POCKET GUIDE TO
NUTRITION AND DIETETICS

This book is dedicated to my family and friends.
Thank you all for your encouragement and support.

SB

For Churchill Livingstone:

Commissioning editor: Ninette Premdas
Project Manager: Derek Robertson
Design Direction: Judith Wright

POCKET GUIDE TO NUTRITION AND DIETETICS

S.E. Byrom BSc(Hons) SRD

Freelance Dietitian, Edinburgh, UK

CHURCHILL
LIVINGSTONE

EDINBURGH LONDON NEW YORK PHILADELPHIA ST LOUIS SYDNEY TORONTO 2002

CHURCHILL LIVINGSTONE
An imprint of Elsevier Limited

First published 2002
    Reprinted 2006

ISBN 0 443 07136 5

British Library Cataloguing in Publication Data
A catalogue record for this book is available from the British Library

Library of Congress Cataloguing in Publication Data
A catalogue record for this book is available from the Library of Congress

Note
Medical knowledge is constantly changing. As new information becomes available,
changes in treatment, procedures, equipment and the use of drugs become
necessary. The author, contributor and the publishers have, as far as it is possible,
taken care to ensure that the information given in this text is accurate and up to date.
However, readers are strongly advised to confirm that the information, especially
with regard to drug usage, complies with the latest legislation and standards of
practice.

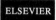

your source for books,
journals and multimedia
in the health sciences

www.elsevierhealth.com

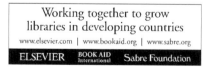

Working together to grow
libraries in developing countries

www.elsevier.com | www.bookaid.org | www.sabre.org

ELSEVIER   BOOK AID International   Sabre Foundation

The
publisher's
policy is to use
paper manufactured
from sustainable forests

Printed in China

Contents

Preface

The first edition of this book, 'The Dietitian's Pocket Book', was written and published by myself. This was a continuation of my final year's honours project as a dietetic student. The book then aimed to provide frequently used clinical data for student dietitians on clinical placement. The second edition still contains a broad range of data but has been thoroughly revised and includes a separate section on paediatric nutritional requirements and information on the new dietetic clinical placement system. The book's broad range of information will appeal to student and qualified dietitians, other health professionals and those interested in the field of nutrition and dietetics. I hope it continues to be a useful pocket guide.

Sarah Byrom BSc (Hons) SRD

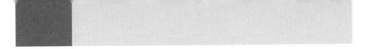

Acknowledgements

I would like to thank everyone who has contributed to the making of this book – all the nutrition companies (listed in Section 4) who helped with the updating of nutritional supplement data, and specifically:

Jacqui Bowden
Head of Clinical Pharmacy, Royal Bournemouth Hospital, Bornemouth

Nicola Glennie
Senior Dietitian, Walsall General Hospital, Birmingham

Dr Patricia Judd
Senior Lecturer in Nutrition & Dietetics, Dietetics Course Organizer, Kings College, London

Rosemarie Simpson-Marks
Education and Training Officer, The British Dietetic Association

Claire Pinder
Paediatric Dietitian, Watford General Hospital, London

Paula Regan
Research Dietitian, Queen Margaret University College, Edinburgh

Janet Smart
Lead Therapist, Royal Infirmary of Edinburgh

Notes – General Guidelines

- This book aims to provide a broad range of data frequently used by dietitians and other healthcare professionals in a clinical setting. Reference ranges and clinical practice will, however, vary among different hospitals, so always follow clinical practice and reference data at the local level.

- Always read through the notes at the beginning of each section before using data. These notes are intended to explain the content of each section, to give further information sources and to list any other considerations specific to each section.

- For queries or further information regarding drugs and nutritional supplements, consult a recent British National Formulary (BNF), Monthly Index of Medical Specialities (MIMS), a clinical pharmacist or manufacturers' drug/nutrition information help lines.

- Medical abbreviations have been used, on occasions, throughout this book. For a full alphabetical listing of these, refer to page 131.

NUTRITIONAL REQUIREMENTS

NOTES

Section 1 is divided into two parts:

- Part 1, Adult Nutritional Requirements
  (covering: basic Anthropometry, Calculation of Adult Nutritional Requirements and Adult Dietary Reference Values (DRVs)).
- Part 2, Paediatric Nutritional Requirements
  (covering: primarily Paediatric DRVs only).

Adult Nutritional Requirements

- Basic adult anthropometry has been outlined at the beginning of this section. This is to enable the reader to calculate body mass index (BMI) and adult energy requirements using the Schofield equation.
- For further anthropometry information, refer to Garrow (2000) and Gibson (1990, 1993). An on-line tutorial is available at Anthropometry Information (refer to p. 140 for the internet address).
- The Schofield equation would normally be used by dietitians as a means of calculating adult energy requirements for enteral tube feeds.
- Further information for the calculation of adult enteral and parenteral nutritional requirements is available from Todorovick & Micklewright (1998).
- For convenience, rich dietary sources of vitamins and minerals have been included among adult DRVs for vitamins and minerals.
- Figures for recommended maximum intakes for alcohol are derived from the Department of Health (1995) and are included at the end of the adult DRVs for convenience.

Paediatric Nutritional Requirements

- This section primarily covers paediatric DRVs only. As these values refer to a 'normal', healthy population, refer to Great

Ormond Street Hospital (2000) for paediatric nutritional requirements for disease states.

- Paediatric normal fluid requirements were derived from Great Ormond Street Hospital (2000). For convenience, these figures are included in the paediatric DRV section.

Definition of Dietary Reference Values (DRVs)

- DRVs have been derived from the report of the COMA Panel on Dietary Reference Values for food energy and nutrients for the United Kingdom (Department of Health 1991). These figures are intended as a guide only and in all cases require individual adaptation based on the individual's nutritional status and dietary intake. DRVs used in Section 1 are defined as follows:

Estimated Average Requirements (EARs)
Estimated average requirement of a group of people for energy. Half of the population usually need more than the EAR, and half less.

Reference Nutrient Intakes (RNIs)
For protein, vitamins or minerals. An amount of a nutrient that is adequate for approximately 97% of the population. The risk of deficiency in this group is very small.

Safe Intakes
In cases where there are insufficient data for nutrients, e.g. for certain vitamins and minerals, safe intakes have been defined. Figures are based on a value which safeguards the individual against deficiency but does not cause any undesirable effects from excess amounts.

Adult Nutritional Requirements

ANTHROPOMETRY

- Anthropometry is the technique of expressing qualitatively the form of the body (Figure 1.1).
- Although there are many anthropometry techniques, height (metres) and weight (kg) are commonly used in clinical

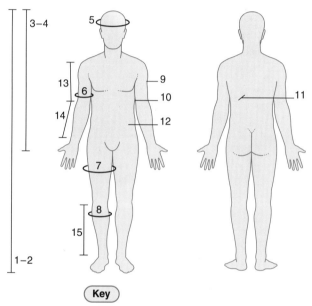

Key

1–2	stature–recumbent length
3–4	sitting height (crown-rump length)
5	head circumference
6	upper-arm circumferences
7	upper-thigh circumferences
8	maximum calf muscle
9	triceps skinfold
10	biceps skinfold
11	subscapular skinfold
12	supra-iliac skinfold
13	upper-arm length
14	forearm length
15	tibial length

Figure 1.1 Anthropometric sites.

practice, since combined they establish a patient's BMI using the BMI equation.

- Body weight is the sum of water, fat, protein, minerals and glycogen.
- Dehydration, ascites, oedema and large surgical amputations will distort weight readings.
- Body fat and lean body tissue can also be measured to reflect nutritional status and body composition. For further details refer to Garrow (2000), Gibson (1990, 1993) and Anthropometry Information (an on-line tutorial; refer to p. 140 for internet address).

Table 1.1 Height conversion table

Feet	Inches	Metres	Feet	Inches	Metres
1	0	0.31	5	5	1.65
2	0	0.61	5	6	1.68
3	0	0.91	5	7	1.70
4	0	1.22	5	8	1.73
4	1	1.25	5	9	1.75
4	2	1.27	5	10	1.78
4	3	1.30	5	11	1.80
4	4	1.32	6	0	1.83
4	5	1.35	6	1	1.85
4	6	1.37	6	2	1.88
4	7	1.40	6	3	1.90
4	8	1.42	6	4	1.93
4	9	1.45	6	5	1.96
4	10	1.47	6	6	1.98
4	11	1.50	6	7	2.01
5	0	1.52	6	8	2.03
5	1	1.55	6	9	2.06
5	2	1.58	6	10	2.08
5	3	1.60	6	11	2.11
5	4	1.63	7	0	2.13

Source: Extracts from British Standards are reproduced with the permission of BSI under licence number 2000SK/0508. Complete standards can be obtained by post from BSI Customer Services, 389 Chiswick High Road, London W4 4AL.

Table 1.2 Weight conversion table

Pounds

Stones	0	1	2	3	4	5	6	7	8	9	10	11	12	13
0		0.45	0.91	1.36	1.81	2.27	2.72	3.18	3.63	4.08	4.54	4.98	5.44	5.89
1	6.35	6.80	7.26	7.71	8.16	8.62	9.07	9.53	9.98	10.43	10.89	11.33	11.79	12.24
2	12.70	13.15	13.61	14.06	14.51	14.97	15.42	15.88	16.33	16.78	17.24	17.68	18.12	18.59
3	19.05	19.50	19.96	20.41	20.86	21.32	21.77	22.23	22.68	23.13	23.59	24.03	24.49	24.94
4	25.40	25.85	26.31	26.76	27.21	27.67	28.12	28.58	28.03	29.48	29.94	30.38	30.84	31.29
5	31.75	32.20	32.66	33.11	33.56	34.02	34.47	34.93	35.38	35.83	36.29	36.73	37.19	37.64
6	38.10	38.55	39.01	39.46	39.91	40.37	40.82	41.28	41.73	42.18	42.64	43.08	43.54	43.99
7	44.45	44.90	45.36	45.81	46.26	46.72	47.17	47.63	48.08	48.53	48.99	49.43	49.89	50.34
8	50.80	51.25	51.71	52.16	52.61	53.07	53.52	53.98	54.43	54.88	55.34	55.78	56.24	56.69
9	57.15	57.60	58.06	58.51	58.96	59.42	59.87	60.33	60.78	61.23	61.69	62.13	62.59	63.04
10	63.50	63.95	64.41	64.86	65.31	65.77	66.22	66.68	67.13	67.58	68.04	68.48	68.94	69.39
11	69.85	70.30	70.76	71.21	71.66	72.12	72.57	73.03	73.48	73.93	74.39	74.83	75.39	75.74
12	76.20	76.65	77.11	77.56	78.01	78.47	78.92	79.38	79.83	80.28	80.74	81.18	81.64	82.09
13	82.55	83.00	83.46	83.91	84.36	84.82	85.27	85.73	86.18	86.63	86.99	87.53	87.99	88.44
14	88.90	89.35	89.81	90.26	90.71	91.17	91.62	92.08	92.53	92.98	93.44	93.88	94.34	94.79
15	95.25	95.70	96.16	96.61	97.06	97.52	97.97	98.43	98.88	99.33	99.79	100.23	100.69	101.14
16	101.60	102.05	102.51	102.96	103.41	103.87	104.32	104.78	105.23	105.68	106.14	106.58	107.04	107.49
17	107.95	108.40	108.86	109.31	109.76	110.22	110.67	111.13	111.58	112.03	112.49	112.93	113.39	113.84
18	114.30	114.75	115.21	115.66	116.11	116.57	117.02	117.48	117.93	118.38	118.84	119.28	119.74	120.19

Source: Extracts from British Standards are reproduced with the permission of BSI under licence number 2000K/0508. Complete standards can be obtained by post from BSI Customer Services, 389 Chiswick High Road, London W4 4AL.

Body Mass Index (BMI) equation

Quetelet index or BMI expresses grades of obesity in adults (refer to BMI equation below and Table 1.3).

$$BMI = \frac{Weight\ (kg)}{Height\ (m^2)}$$

Table 1.3
Grades of obesity

Source: Adapted from Garrow & Webster (1985).

Grade	BMI range	Comments
	<15	Severely underweight
	15–20	Underweight
	20–25	Desirable weight range
1	25–30	Overweight
2	30–40	Very overweight
3	>40	Severely overweight

Table 1.4 Adult desirable weight/height[a] (ready reckoner)

Gender: Male   **Female**

Height (without shoes) (m)	Weight (mean for medium build) (kg)[b]	Height (without shoes) (m)	Weight (mean for medium build) (kg)[b]
1.55	54	1.42	45
1.57	55	1.45	46
1.60	57	1.47	47
1.62	58	1.50	49
1.65	60	1.52	50
1.67	62	1.55	51
1.70	64	1.57	53
1.72	65	1.60	55
1.75	67	1.62	57
1.77	69	1.65	59
1.80	71	1.67	61
1.83	74	1.70	63
1.86	75	1.72	64
1.88	78	1.75	66
1.91	80	1.77	68

Source: Modified from Entwistle (1998).
[a] Figures based on BMIs between 21 and 22 for a medium adult build. Individual BMIs should be calculated using the BMI equation, p. 9.
[b] All weights with indoor clothes, no shoes.

CALCULATING ADULT NUTRITIONAL REQUIREMENTS

Calculating Energy Requirements Using the Schofield Equation

1. Determine the patient's basal metabolic rate (BMR) using the Schofield equation (refer to Table 1.5).

2. To the BMR add:
   a. stress factor (refer to Figure 1.2)
   b. activity and diet-induced thermogenesis
      - Bedbound immobile   +10%
      - Bedbound mobile/sitting   +15–20%
      - Mobile on ward   +25%
   c. add 1672–4180 kJ/day (400–1000 kcal/day) if an increase in energy stores is required. Reduce energy intake if a decrease in energy stores is required.

Source: Adapted from Todorovic & Micklewright (1998).

Table 1.5 Schofield equation[a]

Age (years)	Males	Females
15–18	17.6 W + 656	13.3 W + 690
18–30	15.0 W + 690	14.8 W + 485
30–60	11.4 W + 870	8.1 W + 842
>60	11.7 W + 585	9.0 W + 656

Source: Schofield (1985).
[a] Weight (W) in kg.

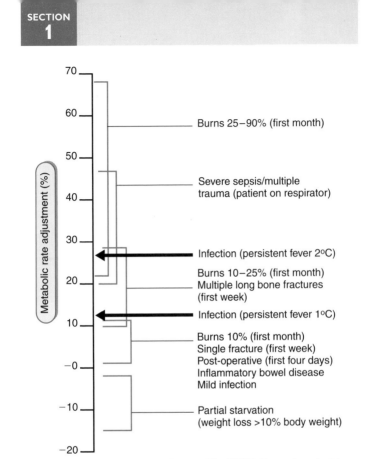

Figure 1.2 Elia Normagram. Source: Elia (1990). Reproduced with permission.

Table 1.6 Guidelines for calculating adult nutritional requirements[a,b]

Metabolic state	Energy (kJ/kg) (kcal/kg)	Protein (g/kg)	Nitrogen (g/kg)	Fluid (ml/kg)	Sodium[c] (mmol/kg)	Potassium (mmol/g nitrogen)	Phosphate (mmol/d)
Normal	105–150 (25–35)	1.0	0.17	30–35	1.0	5.0	20
Intermediate	150–170 (35–40)	1.3–1.9	0.2–0.3	30–35	1.0	5.0	20–30
Hypermetabolic	170–250 (40–60)	2.0–3.0	0.3–0.45	30–35	1.0	7.0	≤50

Source: Main source adapted from Payne-James & Wicks (1994).

[a] Per kg body weight per day, unless otherwise stated.

[b] These figures are intended as guidelines only for selected adult nutritional requirements. Always assess patients on an individual basis and allow provision for non-renal fluid losses (e.g. diarrhoea, fistulas) and pyrexia. For further information, refer to Todorovic & Micklewright (1998).

[c] Allow a minimum of 50 mmol sodium/day.

ADULT DIETARY REFERENCE VALUES

Table 1.7 Adult estimated average requirements (EARs) for energy

Age	EARs MJ/d (kcal/d)	
	Females	**Males**
19–50 years	8.10 (1940)	10.60 (2550)
51–59 years	8.00 (1900)	10.60 (2550)
60–64 years	7.99 (1900)	9.93 (2380)
65–74 years	7.96 (1900)	9.71 (2330)
75+ years	7.61 (1810)	8.77 (2100)
Pregnancy	+0.80[a] (200)	
Lactation		
1 month	+1.90 (450)	
2 months	+2.20 (530)	
3 months	+2.40 (570)	
4–6 months (group 1)[b]	+2.00 (480)	
4–6 months (group 2)[c]	+2.40 (570)	
>6 months (group 1)[b]	+1.00 (240)	
>6 months (group 2)[c]	+2.30 (550)	

Source: © DoH (1991), with permission.
Abbreviations: MJ = megajoule, kcal = kilocalorie.
[a] Last trimester only.
[b] Group 1—women breastfeeding their baby until 3–4 months of age, and thereafter progressively introducing weaning foods.
[c] Group 2—women breastfeeding their baby until 6 months of age or more, whereby breast milk provides the primary source of nourishment.

Table 1.8 Adult reference nutrient intakes for protein

Age	Reference nutrient intake[a] (g/d)	
	Females	**Males**
19–50 years	45.0	55.5
50+	46.5	53.5
Pregnancy[b]	+6	
Lactation[b]		
0–4 months	+11	
4+ months	+8	

Source: © DoH (1991), with permission.
[a] These figures, based on egg and milk protein, assume complete digestibility.
[b] To be added to adult requirements through all stages of pregnancy and lactation.

Table 1.9 Adult dietary reference values for fat and carbohydrate as a percentage of daily energy intake (percentage of food energy)

Energy source	Individual minimum		Population average[a]	Individual maximum
Saturated fatty acids			10 (11)	
Cis-polyunsaturated fatty acids[b]	n-3	0.2	6 (6.5)	10
	n-6	1.0		
Cis-monounsaturated fatty acids			12 (13)	
Trans fatty acids			2 (2)	
Total fatty acids			30 (32.5)	
Total fat			**33 (35)**	
Non-milk extrinsic sugars	0		10 (11)	
Intrinsic and milk sugars and starch			37 (39)	
Total carbohydrate			**47 (50)**	
Non-starch polysaccharide[c] (g/d)	12		**18**	24

Source: Adapted from DoH (1991).

[a] Average figures are given as percentages both of total energy and, in parentheses, of food energy. The average percentage contribution to total energy does not total 100%, as figures for protein and alcohol are excluded.

[b] *Cis*-polyunsaturated fatty acids should be derived from a mixture of n-6 and n-3 polyunsaturated fatty acids (PUFAs).

[c] As non-starch polysaccharides (NSPs) form the major component of plant cell walls, this term is now used instead of 'dietary fibre'.

Table 1.10   Adult reference nutrient intakes for vitamins

Age	Thiamine (mg/d)	Riboflavin (mg/d)	Niacin (nicotinic acid equivalent) (mg/d)	Vitamin B$_6$ (mg/d^a)	Vitamin B$_{12}$ (μg/d)	Folate (μg/d)	Vitamin C (mg/d)	Vitamin A (μg/d)	Vitamin D (μg/d)
Males									
19–50 years	1.0	1.3	17	1.4	1.5	200	40	700	b
50+ years	0.9	1.3	16	1.4	1.5	200	40	700	c
Females									
19–50 years	0.8	1.1	13	1.2	1.5	200	40	600	b
50+ years	0.8	1.1	12	1.2	1.5	200	40	600	c
Pregnancy	+0.1^d	+0.3	e	e	e	+100	+10^d	+100	10
Lactation									
0–4 months	+0.2	+0.5	+2	e	+0.5	+60	+30	+350	10
4+ months	+0.2	+0.5	+2	e	+0.5	+60	+30	+350	10

Source: © DoH (1991), with permission.

^{a} Based on protein providing 14.7% of EAR for energy.

^{b} No DRV for vitamin D is set for adults 18–65 years of age, as solar UV radiation (sunlight) on the skin synthesizes sufficient levels of vitamin D within the body. Individuals with little sunlight exposure may require a vitamin D supplement.

^{c} After age 65 years, the RNI is 10 μg/d for men and women.

^{d} For last trimester only.

^{e} No increment.

Table 1.11 Water-soluble vitamins (rich dietary sources)

Vitamin	Rich dietary sources	Deficiency diseases	Symptoms	Risk groups
C (ascorbic acid)	• citrus fruits • strawberries • nectarines • melons • potatoes • tomatoes	Scurvy	Slow healing of wounds, bleeding gums, loose teeth	Patients who have undergone extensive, repeated surgery. Seriously ill patients with fever. Burns and patients with tumours
B$_1$ (thiamine)	• wheatgerm • wholegrains • yeast • liver • fish • poultry • pork • beans	Beriberi	Muscle paralysis, irritability, fatigue, mental confusion	Alcoholics, persons consuming a refined diet
B$_2$ (riboflavin)	• fortified breakfast cereals • meat • offal • dairy products	Ariboflavinosis	Stomatitis (skin defects around the mouth and nose), corneal vascularization, glossitis	Women who are pregnant or breastfeeding consuming insufficient quantities of dairy products

Table 1.11 Water-soluble vitamins (rich dietary sources)—continued

Vitamin	Rich dietary sources	Deficiency diseases	Symptoms	Risk groups
	• eggs • green leafy vegetables • pulses			Patients with intestinal disease, alcoholics
B$_6$ (pyridoxine)	• fish • poultry • lean meats • wholegrain cereals • nuts • pulses • potatoes • bananas	Anaemia	Listlessness, depression, flaky skin around the nose, mouth and eyes. Poor body growth	Alcoholics, women taking the contraceptive pill and pregnant women
B$_{12}$ (cyanocobalamin)	• offal • meat • oily fish • eggs • dairy products • Barmen • Tastex • Marmite	Pernicious anaemia	Neurological defects	Vegans. Gastrectomy[a] patients

Table 1.11 Water-soluble vitamins (rich dietary sources)—continued

Vitamin	Rich dietary sources	Deficiency diseases	Symptoms	Risk groups
Folic acid (folacin)	• fortified soya milk, fruit drinks and breakfast cereals • offal • meat • dairy products • green leafy vegetables • potatoes • fruit	Anaemia	Inflamed gastrointestinal mucous membrane	Women taking the contraceptive pill and pregnant women. Patients with malabsorption disorders and alcoholics

Source: Adapted from Barasi (1997).

NB: Other water-soluble vitamins include biotin, niacin and pantothenic acid.

[a] Only when an intrinsic factor (produced in the stomach) and an extrinsic factor (contained in the vitamin) combine together can vitamin B_{12} be utilized by the body. Therefore, total gastrectomy patients are likely to suffer from anaemia unless they receive regular vitamin B_{12} injections.

Table 1.12 Fat-soluble vitamins (rich dietary sources)

Vitamin	Rich dietary sources	Deficiency diseases	Symptoms	Risk groups
A (retinol)	• liver • fatty fish • eggs • dairy products • oranges • yellow/green fruit and vegetables	Xerophthalmia (night blindness)	Poor dark adaptation, corneal sores, stunted growth, fatigue	Patients using laxatives, those with poor fat digestion, e.g. cystic fibrosis and pancreatitis
D (cholecalciferol)	• offal • oily fish • egg yolks • full-fat milk and cheese • fortified fat spreads	Rickets	Weak/soft bones (osteomalacia), deformation of bones and teeth, calcium loss from bones	Elderly confined indoors, dark-skinned children, patients with disturbed fat digestion
E (tocopherals)	• offal • eggs • wheatgerm • cereals • nuts • green vegetables • vegetable oils	Anaemia, muscular degeneration (myopathy), reproductive failure, nerve damage	Instability of membrane structures, changes in connective tissue	Patients with poor fat digestion

Table 1.12 Fat-soluble vitamins (rich dietary sources)—continued

Vitamin	Rich dietary sources	Deficiency diseases	Symptoms	Risk groups
K	• liver • dairy products • green leafy vegetables • oils • potatoes • fruits	Reduced haemolysis (reduced blood clotting factor)	Delayed blood coagulation	Newborn babies, patients on antibiotics or medication which affects the intestinal flora, patients on anticoagulant medications, e.g. warfarin

Source: Adapted from Barasi (1997).

Table 1.13 Adult reference nutrient intakes for minerals

Age	Calcium (mg/d)	Phosphorus[a] (mg/d)	Magnesium (mg/d)	Sodium[b] (mg/d)	Potassium[c] (mg/d)	Chloride[d] (mg/d)	Iron (mg/d)	Zinc (mg/d)	Copper (mg/d)	Selenium (µg/d)	Iodine (µg/d)
Males											
19–50 years	700	550	300	1600	3500	2500	8.7	9.5	1.2	75	140
50+ years	700	550	300	1600	3500	2500	8.7	9.5	1.2	75	140
Females											
19–50 years	700	550	270	1600	3500	2500	14.8[e]	7.0	1.2	60	140
50+ years	700	550	270	1600	3500	2500	8.7	7.0	1.2	60	140
Preg-nancy	f	f	f	f	f	f	f	f	f	f	f
Lactation											
0–4 months	+550	+440	+50	f	f	f	f	+6.0	+0.3	+15	f
4+ months	+550	+440	+50	f	f	f	f	+2.5	+0.3	+15	f

Source: © DoH (1991), with permission.

[a] Phosphorus RNI is set equal to calcium in molar terms.
[b] 1 mmol sodium = 23 mg.
[c] 1 mmol potassium = 39 mg.
[d] corresponds to sodium 1 mmol = 35.5 mg.
[e] Insufficient for women with high menstrual losses, where the most practical way of meeting iron requirements is to take an iron supplement.
[f] No increment.

Table 1.14   Minerals (rich dietary sources)

Minerals	Rich dietary sources	Functions
Calcium	• dairy products, fish • fortified soya milk, bread and breakfast cereals • spring cabbage, broccoli • apricots, raisins • almonds, cashew nuts	Strong bones, teeth and muscle tissue. Regulates activity of heart muscle, muscle action, nerve function and blood clotting
Chromium	• meat • wholegrains • brewers' yeast • legumes, nuts	Glucose metabolism (energy), increases effectiveness of insulin
Copper	• oysters, nuts, offal, legumes	Formation of red blood cells, bone growth. Works with vitamin C to form elastin
Iodine	• seafood, sea salt • milk and dairy products	Component of hormone thyroxine, which controls metabolism
Iron	• lean meat, offal, fish, eggs • wholegrain foods, wheatgerm, fortified breakfast cereals • pulses, nuts, seeds, dried fruit • dark green vegetables	Haemoglobin formation, improves blood quality, increases resistance to stress and disease
Magnesium	• wholegrains, nuts, green vegetables	Acid/alkaline balance, important in metabolism of carbohydrates, minerals and sugar
Manganese	• wholegrains, tea, nuts, fruit and vegetables	Enzyme activations, carbohydrate and fat production, sex hormone production, skeletal development
Phosphorus	• meat, poultry, fish, eggs, cereal products	Bone development, important in protein, fat and carbohydrate utilization
Potassium	• meat, pork, fish, fruit, potatoes, beans, dried peas	Fluid balance, controls activity of heart muscle, nervous system and kidneys
Selenium	• lean meats, offal, seafood, eggs, wholegrains	Protects body tissues against oxidative radiation, pollution and normal metabolic processing

Table 1.14 Minerals (rich dietary sources)—continued

Minerals	Rich dietary sources	Functions
Zinc	• lean meats, liver, seafood, eggs, cheese	Involved in digestion and metabolism, important in the development of the reproductive system, aids in wound healing

Source: Adapted from Barasi (1997).

Table 1.15 Adult safe intakes for vitamins and minerals

Nutrient	Safe intake
Vitamins	
Pantothenic acid	3–7 mg/d
Biotin	10–200 µg/d
Vitamin E	
Men	Above 4 mg/d
Women	Above 3 mg/d
Vitamin K	1 µg/kg/d
Minerals	
Manganese	Above 1.4 mg/d (26 µmol/d)
Molybdenum	50–400 µg/d
Chromium	Above 25 µg (0.5 µmol/d)
Fluoride	0.5 mg/kg/d (3 µmol/kg/d)

Source: Adapted from DoH (1991).

Recommended Maximum Intakes for Alcohol (Department of Health 1995)

Recommended maximum intakes:

- women 2–3 units/day (14–21 units/week)
- men 3–4 units/day (21–28 units/week)

1 unit of alcohol is equivalent to:

- half a pint of ordinary beer, lager or cider
- one single pub measure of spirits (whisky, gin, bacardi, vodka)

- one standard glass of wine (125 ml)
- one small glass of sherry
- one measure of vermouth or aperitif

Gill measures:
- England/Wales = 1/6 gill
- Northern Ireland = 1/4 gill
- Scotland = 1/5 or 1/4 gill

NB: Owing to a lower percentage of body water composition, women are at a greater risk of the harmful effects of alcohol than men (i.e. alcohol is absorbed in a more concentrated form in women compared to men).

Paediatric Nutritional Requirements

Table 1.16 Paediatric weight ranges for the UK population (0–19 years) (male/female 2nd, 50th and 98th centiles for weight)

Age	Males			Females		
	2nd centile	50th centile	98th centile	2nd centile	50th centile	98th centile
0 month	2.7	3.6	4.7	2.6	3.4	4.3
3 months	4.9	6.3	7.8	4.7	5.7	7.3
6 months	6.5	8.1	9.9	6.2	7.5	9.3
9 months	7.4	9.2	11.4	7.0	8.6	10.6
12 months	8.2	10.2	12.5	7.7	9.5	11.7
1.5 years	9.3	11.4	14.2	8.8	10.8	13.5
2.0 years	10.1	12.5	15.6	9.7	12.0	15.0
2.5 years	10.9	13.5	17.0	10.5	13.0	17.0
3.0 years	11.8	14.7	18.5	11.3	14.0	18.2
3.5 years	12.6	15.6	19.8	12.0	15.0	19.5
4.0 years	13.3	16.5	21.1	13.0	16.0	21.5
4.5 years	14.0	17.5	22.5	13.5	17.0	23.0
5.0 years	14.8	18.6	24.2	14.0	18.0	24.5

Table 1.16 Paediatric weight ranges for UK population (0–19 years) (male/female 2nd, 50th and 98th centiles for weight)—continued

Age	Males			Females		
	2nd centile	50th centile	98th centile	2nd centile	50th centile	98th centile
5.5 years	15.8	20.0	26.0	15.0	19.4	26.5
6.5 years	17.4	22.0	29.5	16.5	21.5	30.0
7.5 years	19.0	24.4	33.5	18.2	24.2	35.0
8.5 years	21.0	27.0	39.0	20.2	27.2	40.4
9.5 years	23.0	30.0	44.0	22.3	30.5	46.0
10.5 years	25.0	33.0	49.5	24.5	34.0	52.5
11.5 years	27.0	36.5	55.0	27.0	38.0	58.0
12.5 years	29.5	40.2	61.0	30.2	42.8	63.0
13.5 years	32.8	46.0	68.0	34.7	48.0	68.0
14.5 years	37.0	52.0	77.0	38.5	52.0	72.0
15.5 years	42.0	58.0	83.5	41.5	54.5	74.8
16.5 years	47.0	62.5	87.2	43.0	56.2	76.7
17.5 years+	52.0	67.0	90.5	44.0	57.0	78.0

Source: Data compiled by GOSH (2000). Data obtained using male and female growth charts (birth to 18 years), published by the Child Growth Foundation, 1996. Copies of the growth charts available from: Child Growth Foundation, 2 Mayfield Avenue, London W4 1PW.

PAEDIATRIC DIETARY REFERENCE VALUES

Table 1.17 Paediatric estimated average requirements (EAR) for energy

Age	EARs MJ/d (kcal/d)	
	Males	**Females**
0–3 months	2.28 (545)	2.16 (515)
4–6 months	2.89 (690)	2.69 (645)
7–9 months	3.44 (825)	3.2 (765)
10–12 months	3.85 (920)	3.61 (865)
1–3 years	5.15 (1230)	4.86 (1165)
4–6 years	7.16 (1715)	6.46 (1545)
7–10 years	8.24 (1970)	7.28 (1740)
11–14 years	9.27 (2220)	7.72 (1845)
15–18 years	11.51 (2775)	8.83 (2110)

Source: © DoH (1991), with permission.
Abbreviations: MJ = megajoule, kcal = kilocalorie.

Table 1.18 Paediatric reference nutrient intakes for protein

Age	Reference nutrient intake[a] (g/d)
0–3 months	12.5[b]
4–6 months	12.7
7–9 months	13.7
10–12 months	14.9
1–3 years	14.5
4–6 years	19.7
7–10 years	28.3
Males	
11–14 years	42.1
15–18 years	55.2
Females	
11–14 years	41.2
15–18 years	45.0

Source: © DoH (1991), with permission.
[a] These figures, based on egg and milk protein, assume complete digestibility.
[b] No values for infants 0–3 months are given by the World Health Organization. The RNI is calculated by the recommendations of the Committee on Medical Aspects of Food Policy (COMA).

Table 1.19 Paediatric normal fluid requirements

Age/Weight (kg)	Approximate weight (kg)	Fluid[a] (ml/kg)
Premature	1–2	150–200
0–6 months	2–8	150
7–12 months	6–10	120
Children weighing over 11–20 kg	–	100 ml/kg for the first 10 kg +50 ml/kg for the next 10 kg
Children weighing 20 kg and above	–	100 ml/kg for the first 10 kg +50 ml/kg for the next 10 kg +25 ml/kg thereafter (up to 2500 ml maximum per day)

Source: © GOSH Dietetic Department (2000), with permission.
NB: These ranges are intended as guidelines only. Allow provisions for pyrexia, hot weather and increased physical activity.
[a] Overweight children will require less fluid than the calculated volume. For underweight children, calculate fluid requirements per child's actual weight (but an increase in energy/protein intake may be required for 'catch-up' growth).

Table 1.20 Paediatric dietary reference values for fat and carbohydrate

Energy source	Requirements
Saturated fatty acids	11% of total dietary energy
Cis-monounsaturated fatty acids	13% of total dietary energy (principally oleic acid)
Cis-polyunsaturated fatty acids	6.5% of total dietary energy to a maximum of 10% including:
• Linoleic acid	≥1% total dietary energy
• Alpha-linoleic acid	≥0.2% total dietary energy
Trans fatty acids	No greater than 2% of total dietary energy
Total fatty acid intake	33% (average figure) and total fat intake 35% of total dietary energy
Non-milk extrinsic sugar	No greater than 11% of total dietary energy (infant formulae should contain 40% of energy from lactose)
Starch	39% of total dietary energy (with intrinsic and milk sugars) for adults and children over 2 years
Non-starch polysaccharide (NSP)[a]	No specific recommendations for children

Source: © DoH (1991) (data derived from). © GOSH Dietetic Department (2000) (data compiled by), with permission.

[a] As NSP forms the major component of plant cell walls, it is now used as the single index for the term 'dietary fibre'. Children under 2 years should not be given NSP-rich foods when more energy-dense foods are required.

Table 1.21 Paediatric reference nutrient intakes for vitamins

Age	Thiamine (mg/d)	Riboflavin (mg/d)	Niacin (nicotinic acid equivalent) (mg/d)	Vitamin B$_6$[a] (mg/d)	Vitamin B$_{12}$ (µg/d)	Folate (µg/d)	Vitamin C (mg/d)	Vitamin A (µg/d)	Vitamin D[b] (µg/d)
0–3 months	0.2	0.4	3	0.2	0.3	50	25	350	8.5
4–6 months	0.2	0.4	3	0.2	0.3	50	25	350	8.5
7–9 months	0.2	0.4	4	0.3	0.4	50	25	350	7
10–12 months	0.3	0.4	5	0.4	0.4	50	25	350	7
1–3 years	0.5	0.6	8	0.7	0.5	70	30	400	7
4–6 years	0.7	0.8	11	0.9	0.8	100	30	400	b
7–10 years	0.7	1.0	12	1.0	1.0	150	30	500	b
Males									
11–14 years	0.9	1.2	15	1.2	1.2	200	35	600	b
15–18 years	1.1	1.3	18	1.5	1.5	200	40	700	b
Females									
11–14 years	0.7	1.1	12	1.0	1.2	200	35	600	b
15–18 years	0.8	1.1	14	1.2	1.5	200	40	600	b

Source: © DoH (1991), with permission.

[a] Based on protein providing 14.7% of EAR for energy.

[b] No DRV for vitamin D is set for ages 4–18 years, as solar UV radiation (sunlight) on the skin synthesizes sufficient levels of vitamin D within the body. Individuals with little sunlight exposure may require a vitamin D supplement.

Table 1.22 Paediatric reference nutrient intakes for minerals

Age	Calcium (mg/d)	Phosphorus[a] (mg/d)	Magnesium (mg/d)	Sodium[b] (mg/d)	Potassium[c] (mg/d)	Chloride[d] (mg/d)	Iron (mg/d)	Zinc (mg/d)	Copper (mg/d)	Selenium (µg/d)	Iodine (µg/d)
0–3 months	525	400	55	210	800	320	1.7	4.0	0.2	10	50
4–6 months	525	400	60	280	850	400	4.3	4.0	0.3	13	60
7–9 months	525	400	75	320	700	500	7.8	5.0	0.3	10	60
10–12 months	525	400	80	350	700	500	7.8	5.0	0.3	10	60
1–3 years	350	270	85	500	800	800	6.9	5.0	0.4	15	70
4–6 years	450	350	120	700	1100	1100	6.1	6.5	0.6	20	100
7–10 years	550	450	200	1200	2000	1800	8.7	7.0	0.7	30	110
Males											
11–14 years	1000	775	280	1600	3100	2500	11.3	9.0	0.8	45	130
15–18 years	1000	775	300	1600	3500	2500	11.3	9.5	1.0	70	140
Females											
11–14 years	800	625	280	1600	3100	2500	14.8[e]	9.0	0.8	45	130
15–18 years	800	625	300	1600	3500	2500	14.8[e]	7.0	1.0	60	140

Source: © DoH (1991), with permission.

[a] Phosphorus RNI is set equal to calcium in molar terms.

[b] 1 mmol sodium = 23 mg.

[c] 1 mmol potassium = 39 mg.

[d] Corresponds to sodium 1 mmol = 35.3 mg.

[e] Insufficent for females with high menstrual losses, where the most practical way of meeting iron requirements is to take an iron supplement.

Table 1.23 Paediatric safe intakes for vitamins and minerals

Nutrient	Age group	Safe intake
Vitamins		
Pantothenic acid	Infants	1.7 mg/d
Biotin	–	10–200 µg/d
Vitamin E	Infants	0.4 mg/g polyun-saturated fatty acids
Vitamin K	Infants	10 µg/d
Minerals		
Manganese	Infants and children	Above 16 µg (0.3 µmol)/kg/d
Molybdenum	Infants, children and adolescents	0.5–1.5 µg/kg/d
Chromium	Children and adolescents	0.1–1.0 µg (2–20 nmol)/kg/d
Fluoride	Infants under 6 months	0.22 mg/kg/d (12 µmol/kg/d)
	Children over 6 months	0.12 mg/kg/d (6 µmol/kg/d)
	Children over 6 years	0.5 mg/kg/d (3 µmol/kg/d)

Source: Adapted from DoH (1991).

Table 1.24 Weaning guide[a]

Age group	Milk	Dairy produce and substitutes	Starchy foods	Fruit and vegetables	Meat and meat alternatives
4–6 months	Minimum 600 ml breast or infant formula milk daily	Cow's milk products (e.g. yoghurt, custard, cheese sauce)	Mix smooth cereal with milk; use low-fibre cereals (e.g. rice-based). Mash or puree starchy vegetables (e.g. potatoes), rusks and baby rice	Mash or puree (removing pips and core), e.g. bananas, pears	Soft-cooked meat/ pulses (avoid adding salt or sugar)
6–9 months	500–600 ml breast milk, infant formula or follow-on formula daily	Milk[b] to mix solids. Hard cheese (e.g. cheddar) cubed or grated	2–3 servings daily Start to introduce some wholemeal bread and cereals. Foods can have a more solid 'lumpier' texture. Begin to give 'finger foods' (e.g. toast) and bread sticks	2 servings daily Raw soft fruit and vegetables (e.g. banana, melon, tomato) may be used as 'finger foods.' Cooked vegetables and fruit can be of a coarser, mashed texture	1 serving daily Soft-cooked minced or pureed meat/ fish/pulses. Chopped hard-boiled eggs can be used as a 'finger food'
9–12 months	500–600 ml breast milk or infant formula milk daily	Milk[b] to mix solids, hard cheese cubed or grated	3–4 servings daily Starchy foods can be of normal adult texture.	3–4 servings daily Encourage lightly cooked or raw fruit and vegetables	Minimum 1 serving daily from animal source or 2 from

Table 1.24 Weaning guide[a]—continued

Age group	Milk	Dairy produce and substitutes	Starchy foods	Fruit and vegetables	Meat and meat alternatives	vegetable sources
			Encourage wholemeal products	are rejected. Chopped or 'finger food' texture is suitable. Unsweetened orange juice with meals, especially if diet is meat-free		In a vegetarian diet, use a mixture of different vegetables and starchy foods (macaroni cheese, dhal and rice)
After 1 year	Minimum 350 ml milk daily or two servings of dairy products (e.g. yoghurt, cheese sauce)	Whole milk can be used as a drink (lower-fat milks can be used in cooking, but not as main drink). Soft cheeses	**Minimum of 4 servings daily** At least one serving at each mealtime. Discourage high-fat foods (crisps, savoury snacks and pastry)	**Minimum 4 servings daily** Encourage unsweetened pies and stews. Vegetables may be preferred raw (e.g. grated carrot, chopped tomato) or may need to be disguised in soups, pies and stews	**Minimum 1 serving daily from animal source or 2 from vegetable source** Encourage low-fat meat and oily fish (sardine, herring and mackerel). Liver pate may also be used	

[a] For a normal, healthy baby.

[b] Includes breast milk, infant formula, follow-on formula and whole cow's milk.

NB: Breast milk, whenever possible, should always be encouraged, in preference to formula milks.

REFERENCES

Barasi ME (1997)
Human nutrition: a health perspective, 1st edn. London: Arnold.

Department of Health (1991)
Report on health and social subjects. No. 41. Dietary reference values for food energy and nutrients for the United Kingdom COMA. London: HMSO.

Department of Health (1995)
Drinking sensibly: a discussion document. London: HMSO. (Currently out of print. Copies may be available from the Department of Health, London, or academic libraries specializing in the field of nutrition and dietetics.)

Elia M (1990)
Artificial nutritional support. Med Int 82: 3392–3396.

Entwistle IR (1998)
Exacta medica: reference tables and data for the medical and nursing professions, 2nd edn. Edinburgh: Churchill Livingstone.

Garrow JS (2000)
Composition of the body. In: Garrow JS, James WPT, Ralph A, eds. Human nutrition and dietetics, 10th edn. Edinburgh: Churchill Livingstone: 13–23.

Garrow JS, Webster J (1985)
Quetelet's index (w/h^2) as a measure of fatness. Int J Obesity 9: 147–153.

Gibson RS (1990)
Principles of nutritional assessment. New York: Oxford University Press.

Gibson RS (1993)
Nutritional assessment: a laboratory manual. New York: Oxford University Press.

Great Ormond Street Hospital (2000)
Nutritional requirements for children in health and disease, 3rd edn. London: Dietetic Department, Great Ormond Street Hospital for Children NHS Trust.

Payne-James J, Wicks C (1994)
Key facts in clinical nutrition, 1st edn. Edinburgh: Churchill Livingstone.

Schofield WN (1985)
Predicting basal metabolic rate, new standards and reviews of previous work. Hum Nutr Clin Nutr 39C: 5–41.

Todorovic VE, Micklewright A (eds) (1998)
A pocket guide to clinical nutrition, 2nd edn, revised. Birmingham: Parenteral and Enteral Nutrition Group of The British Dietetic Association.

ARTIFICIAL NUTRITIONAL SUPPORT

NOTES

- This section aims to provide a brief overview of enteral tube feeding and parenteral nutrition. For further information refer to Payne-James et al (2001), Thomas (2001) and Todorvick & Micklewright (1998).

- Specific standards and guidelines for nutritional support are outlined in McAtear & Wright (1996) and Sizer (1996).

- Although parenteral nutrition (PN) is outlined in this section, student dietitians and most basic-grade dietitians would not be expected to manage PN patients. Students would, however, be expected to have a basic knowledge and understanding of PN.

- Section 4 lists nutritional data for enteral tube feeds (intravenous nutrition solutions for PN may be found in any current British National Formulary).

- Nutrition support teams play a primary role in managing hospital nutritional support. As this area is not described in any detail here, refer to Silk (1994) for further information.

Enteral Tube Feeding

DEFINITION (Reilly 1998)

- Utilizing the gut for the digestion of nutrients administered by an enteral feeding tube.
- May be used for patients who have a functioning gut but insufficient dietary intake, e.g. for 5–7 days or more, or for those unable to meet their nutritional requirements from oral dietary intake alone.

(Refer to Figure 2.1 for anatomy of the gastrointestinal (GI) tract and Table 2.1 for nutrient absorption sites in the GI tract.)

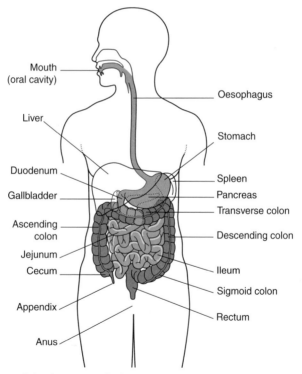

Figure 2.1 Anatomy of the gastrointestinal tract (adapted from Tortora and Grabowski, 1999).

Table 2.1 Nutrient absorption sites in the gastrointestinal (GI) tract

GI site	Nutrient(s) absorbed	Comments
Stomach	None	B_{12} intrinsic factor present
Duodenum	Minerals	Most minerals are absorbed at this point
	Monosaccharides, disaccharides, fatty acids, vitamins A and D, water and sodium	Only small amounts of remaining nutrients (except for water and sodium) absorbed here
Jejunum	Water, sodium, monosaccharides and disaccharides, vitamins A and D, fatty acids, amino acids and simple peptides, water-soluble vitamins	Most water-soluble vitamins, amino acids and simple peptides, disaccharides and water/sodium absorbed at this point
Ileum	Bile salts, vitamin B_{12}, water/sodium, amino acids and simple peptides, water-soluble vitamins	All vitamin B_{12} absorbed and most of the bile salts
Colon	Water/sodium, vitamin K and potassium	Vitamin K formed by bacterial action

Main source: adapted from Whitney et al (1998).

INDICATIONS AND ADMINISTRATION
(McAtear 1999, Reilly 1998)

(Refer to Figure 2.2.)

Short Term

Nasogastric (refer to Figure 2.3)

- For patients who have full use of their stomach with no complications associated with nausea, vomiting or aspiration.

Orogastric

- Used in head injury patients when the extent of damage is unknown (i.e. when there is risk of a nasogastric tube entering the intercranial space if it were passed). It may also

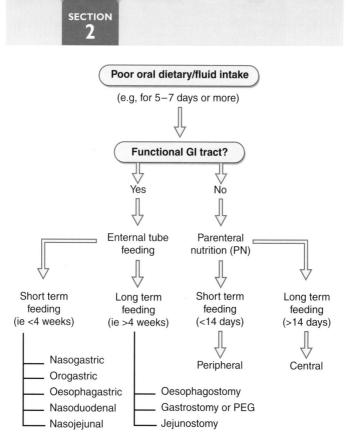

Figure 2.2 Administration and indications for artificial nutritional support.

be used for patients with nasal trauma. However, it is rarely used now, since it is uncomfortable for the patient and may cause dry mouth and ulcerated lips.

Oesophagastric

- Used for head and neck patients. Involves placing a fine-bore tube through the tracheostomy and an existing tracheo-oesophageal fistula.

Nasoduodenal

- For patients requiring their stomach to be bypassed. It is rarely used now, as patients with nausea, vomiting and/or

Nasogastric feeding   **Nasojejunal feeding**

Figure 2.3   Position of nasogastric and nasojejunal feeding tubes.

aspiration usually require enteral tube feeding further down the gut, i.e. into the jejunum, where these symptoms are less likely to persist.

Nasojejunal (refer to Figure 2.3)

- For patients who require both their stomach and duodenum to be bypassed, e.g. patients at risk of aspiration, continual nausea, vomiting and upper GI strictures, obstructions or surgery.

Long Term

Oesophagostomy (Cervical Pharynx)

- Primarily used by surgeons operating on the head and neck. Also known as cervical pharynx. A fine-bore tube is placed surgically through the neck into the oesophagus or pharynx.

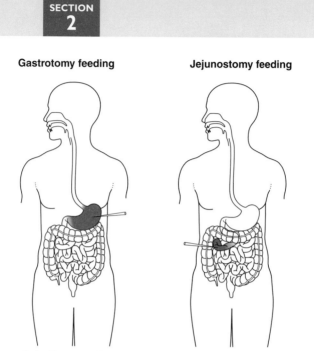

Gastrotomy feeding

Jejunostomy feeding

Figure 2.4 Position of gastrostomy and jejunostomy feeding tubes.

Gastrostomy (refer to Figure 2.4)

- Gastrostomies may be surgically or percutaneously (PEG) placed. A surgically placed gastrostomy requires a general anaesthetic and laparotomy, while a PEG is placed endoscopically under sedation using specially designed kits.

Jejunostomy (refer to Figure 2.4)

- For patients who require both the stomach and duodenum to be bypassed.

Conditions indicating enteral tube feeding may include:

- dysphagic patients
- coma/unconscious patients
- patients with increased nutritional requirements unable to be met by dietary intake alone (e.g. burns, trauma, orthopaedic, HIV and surgical patients)
- early feeding of low-birthweight infants

- chemo/radiotherapy patients
- surgical patients (especially head and neck involvement resulting in physical eating problems)
- depressed patients with prolonged disinterest in food
- dementia patients.

CONTRAINDICATIONS (McAtear 1999)

- Paralytic ileus (absolute contraindication).
- Intestinal obstruction or mobility disorders.
- Any gastrointestinal surgery (pre- and postoperatively) requiring total bowel rest.
- Certain bowel fistulas.
- Acute pancreatitis (although nasojejunal feeding past the pancreas may be suitable).
- Total blockage of the oesophagus.
- When passing an endoscope on the patient is not possible (for PEG patients).

FEEDING TUBES

Wide-bore Nasogastric Tubes (Ryles and Levin's tubes)

- Originally designed for stomach drainage.
- Uncomfortable for patient.
- Can cause oesophageal ulceration.
- Occasionally used for patients at risk of aspiration (e.g. dysphagic patients) or after surgery where there is concern regarding gastric function.

Fine-bore Nasogastric Tubes

- Now most commonly used, since their range of narrow gauges (diameters) and pliability make them more comfortable.
- Available in PVC for short-term feeding, and in polyurethane/silicone for longer-term feeding.
- Guidewires help to administer the passing of a nasogastric tube.

METHODS OF FEED ADMINISTRATION

Bolus Feeding

- 'Infusing' volumes of feed in a feeding tube using a syringe.

- May be used for restless or agitated patients who frequently disconnect 'giving sets' (equipment used to attach feed to pump) or patients who require part infusion feeding to supplement oral dietary intake.

- Now rarely used, as rapid administration of large volumes of feed is associated with diarrhoea and abdominal discomfort.

- If used, a maximum of 250–300 ml of feed is recommended per infusion.

Gravity Feeding

- Continual drip feeding (by adjusting roller clamp on the giving set).

- Drip rate is calculated and adjusted to correspond with the prescribed volume of feed in a set time.

- More time-consuming and less accurate than pump feeding.

Pump Feeding

- Feeding pump controls feed rate.

- Variety of pumps available (including compact ambulatory ones).

- Now most commonly used.

INITIATING ENTERAL TUBE FEEDING

(The following pathway is an example only. Always follow the practice of your own hospital.)

1 Liaise with the medical team.

2 Read through and summarize relevant medical details of the patient.

3 Assess the patient's blood biochemistry (e.g. sodium, potassium, urea, creatinine and albumin) and other parameters such as bowel movement and fluid balance.

4 Nutritionally assess the patient (including nutritional status and dietary intake).

5 Decide if short- or long-term enteral tube feeding is required.

6 Determine the most appropriate route for feed administration.

7 Calculate nutritional requirements.

8 Decide on the most suitable enteral feed to use and volume required.

9 Devise an appropriate feeding regimen.

10 Explain and discuss with nursing staff the devised feeding regimen.

11 Document the dietary assessment and prescription in medical/nursing (or unitary) and dietetic records (leaving a record of the feeding regimen at ward level).

12 Record patient feed details in the dietetic department, as required.

13 Ensure that all enteral feeding equipment and feed is supplied (e.g. feeding pump, feeding tube, giving set and feed).

FEEDING REGIMENS

To devise an enteral tube feeding regimen:

1 Calculate nutritional requirements (based on nutritional assessment of patient).

2 Decide on the most suitable route of administration, feed and extra fluid (as required).

3 Calculate the pump/drip rate for total feed/fluid required over 24 h.

4 Devise regimen.

Patient name .... Type of feed 1500 mls standard 1 kcal/ml .....

Ward .... Type of tube ....

Date	Volume of feed/mls (total 1500 mls)	Delivery rate (mls/hr)	Total feeding time (hrs)	Rest period (hrs)
Day 1	200	50*	4	
	300	75	4	
	500	100	5	
	500	125	4	7
Day 2	1500	125	12	12
Day 3 (established regimen)	1500	150	10	10.5

Finishing

Flush with .... ml sterile water at the beginning and end of feeding and between bottles/bags

Fluid regimes/flushes may be written within the feeding regimen as well. (giving set should be changed every 24 hours)

* If patient has had a prolonged period of starvation prior to feeding start feed rate at 25 mls/hr.

NB: The above is intended as a guide only. Each patient should be individually assessed and reviewed accordingly.

Figure 2.5 Example of a 1500 kcal enteral tube feeding regimen.

Figures 2.5 and 2.6 provide two examples of enteral tube feeding regimens. However, these will vary greatly, depending on the individual patient and style of regimens used by your hospital.

CONSIDERATIONS

• Aim to provide the easiest and most practical feeding regimen for both patient and nurses/carers, accounting for times when a patient may need to be free and ambulatory from their feed, e.g. when leaving a ward to receive physiotherapy/tests.

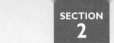

Patient name .... Type of feed 2000 mls standard 1 kcal/ml ....

Ward .... Type of tube ....

Date	Volume of feed/mls (total 2000 mls)	Delivery rate (mls/hr)	Total feeding time (hrs)	Rest period (hrs)
Day 1	200	50*	4	
	300	75	4	
	500	100	5	
	500	125	4	7
Day 2	2000	125	16	12
Day 3 (established regimen)	2000	150	13.5	10.5

Finishing

Flush with .... ml sterile water at the beginning and end of feeding
and between bottles/bags

Fluid regimes/flushes may be written within the feeding regimen as well.
(giving set should be changed every 24 hours)

* If patient has had a prolonged period of starvation prior to feeding
start feed rate at 25 mls/hr.

NB: The above is intended as a guide only. Each patient should be
individually assessed and reviewed accordingly.

Figure 2.6 Example of a 2000 kcal enteral tube feeding regimen.

- When feeding into the stomach, allow at least 6 hours rest per 24 h. During feeding, the pH of the stomach rises. A resting period allows the stomach to return to its normal pH of 2. This helps kill any bacteria present and prevents transmission of gastric organisms to the tracheobronchial tree, reducing the risk of pneumonia.

- For new patients receiving enteral tube feeding, increase the rate of feed gradually (especially for post-gastric feeding), e.g. at intervals of 25 ml/h. Include administration of extra fluid (as required) and water flushes.

- Be aware that feeding pumps may get switched off accidentally or be set at the incorrect rate. Check that the actual feed and feeding rate administered to the patient correspond to the prescribed feeding regimen.
- Ensure that giving sets are changed daily and feeding tubes are flushed before and after feed administration.

MONITORING
(Adapted from Todorvick & Micklewright 1998)

Example checklist for monitoring enteral tube feeding:

- general patient's wellbeing, i.e. tolerance to feed
- regular weights (ideally every 2–3 days) to assess weight gain/ loss
- daily urea and electrolytes
- daily fluid balance
- daily bowel movement to observe any diarrhoea or constipation
- daily dietary intake if applicable (either by taking a 24-h diet history or from food charts)
- blood glucose
- weekly anthropometry (e.g. skin fold thickness)
- other blood results and investigations as indicated (e.g. vitamin and mineral status, liver function test and urinalysis).

COMPLICATIONS (McAtear 1999)

- Refer to Table 2.2 for complications and suggested remedies associated with enteral tube feeding.

Gastrostomy feeding:

- local wound infection
- granulation of tissue
- necrotizing fascites
- intra-abdominal abscesses.

Table 2.2 Complications associated with enteral tube feeding

Complication	Comments	Suggested remedies
Abnormal LFTs	Causes are multifactorial and relate to underlying disease or malnutrition	• Seldom clinically significant in patients without liver disease, so rarely requires cessation of feed
Aspiration	Commonly caused by tube misplacement, delayed gastric emptying or poor gag reflex	• Check tube position (by X-ray or aspiration of gastric acid) • Aspirate tube 4–6-hourly • Wide-bore tube • Elevate patient's head (to a minimum 30° angle) • Reduce gastric motility using antiemetics (see Table 3.9) • If NG feeding, try nasojejunal feeding if continual problem
Constipation	Patients may not be receiving sufficient fluids and/or fibre	• Extra fluid • Consider fibre-containing feed • Appropriate enema, laxatives or bulking agents (see Table 3.6)
Diarrhoea	Rapid feeding rates, bolus feeding and some antibiotics may cause diarrhoea Common in patients fed jejunally Check that this is not an 'overflow' from constipation	• Send a stool sample for culture (to determine any microbial causes) • Anti-diarrhoea agents (see Table 3.4) • Reduce feeding rate/osmolarity • Reduce range of antibiotics if possible • Consider fibre-containing or lactose-free feed
Hyperglycaemia	Usually related to insulin resistance	• Insulin. Aim for continuous feeding to help maintain blood sugar control • Regular monitoring of blood glucose, 4-hourly initially until blood sugars stabilize (see Table 3.3)

Table 2.2 Complications associated with enteral tube feeding—continued

Complication	Comments	Suggested remedies
Tube blockage	Continual feeding at very slow rates (e.g. 10 ml/h) may cause this and additions of medications and/or reconstituted feeds. Regular flushing of tube with sterile water should prevent this	• Flush tube with sterile water mixed with a pinch of sodium bicarbonate, or flush with pancreatic enzyme solution/ diet cola/cranberry or pineapple juice • If administering drugs via feeding tube, ensure they are finely crushed, in liquid form/syrup, and that the tube is flushed well before and after drug administration
Tube withdrawal	Short-term feeding tubes may be pulled out by patients by accident. Others may persistently refuse to keep them down	• If NG feeding, tape the tube securely to the patient's face • If persistently a problem, consider long-term feeding routes
Hyper/hypokalaemia, hyper/hyponatraemia, hyper/hypophosph- ataemia	Renal/liver patients susceptible	• Adjust diet/or enteral feed accordingly, use of 'specialist feeds' as appropriate • Regular monitoring of blood biochemistry • Sodium and/or potassium supplements if very low levels

Main source: adapted from McAtear (1999).
LFT = liver function test; NG = nasogastric.

HOME ENTERAL NUTRITION
(Howard 2000, Schneider et al 2000)

This is an expanding area involving:

- multidisciplinary team approach
- comprehensive patient education
- delivery of feeding equipment and supplies
- home storage of feed and equipment
- domestic disposal of feed and equipment
- provision of follow-up nutrition care
- psychosocial aspects.

DISCHARGE INFORMATION

When a new patient is discharged home from hospital on an enteral tube feed, a dietitian will normally:

- Liaise with nutrition support team members (NST), if applicable, regarding patient/carer education for managing enteral tube feeding at home. An NST member (not necessarily a dietitian, e.g. a nutrition nurse) may have a designated role in doing this. In other cases, the dietitian or a representative from a nutrition company (responsible for providing the feed/equipment) may do this.

- Contact the patient's GP to update them on their patient's current care and feed prescription requirements. (Although most feeds are available on prescription, feeding equipment is not and has to be financed from a hospital or community budget.)

- Liaise with nutrition companies to coordinate the delivery of feeds/equipment, ensuring that a feeding pump is available for the patient to take home. (Carers and relatives may initially require a 24-h telephone help line, which is provided by some nutrition companies.)

- Contact the community dietitian (if applicable), who will continue dietetic care for the patient following discharge.

- Register the patient on the British Artificial Nutrition Survey (BANS) (a home enteral feeding register monitoring aspects of care which vary among different health authorities).
- For further information regarding home enteral feeding, refer to Howard (2000) and Schneider et al (2000).

Parenteral Nutrition

DEFINITION (Pennington 1996)

- The delivery of nutrients directly into the circulatory system using peripheral or central venous access (Figure 2.7). Also known as intravenous (i.v.) feeding.

- The term 'parenteral nutrition' is more accurate to use than 'total parenteral nutrition', as patients may be fed by a combination of both enteral and parenteral routes.

INDICATIONS (Henry 1997)

Absolute Indication

- Non-functioning gut.

Peripheral Parenteral Nutrition

Indicated for patients requiring i.v. feeding for less than 14 days. Most patients requiring parenteral nutrition will

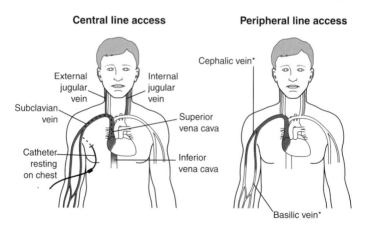

Central line access

External jugular vein

Internal jugular vein

Subclavian vein

Superior vena cava

Catheter resting on chest

Inferior vena cava

Peripheral line access

Cephalic vein*

Basilic vein*

* Access points for catheter (long line) peripheral feeding.
Peripheral feeding using a cannula device may be administered through any vein

Figure 2.7 Parenteral nutrition access routes.

receive peripheral parenteral nutrition (PPN). Conditions indicating PPN include:

- major gastro/excisional surgery requiring total bowel rest pre- and postoperatively
- severe pancreatitis
- mucositis following chemotherapy
- inflammatory bowel disease (e.g. Crohn's disease and ulcerative colitis)
- multiorgan failure (when nutritional requirements cannot be met by enteral nutrition alone)
- enterocutaneous fistulas.

Central Line Parenteral Nutrition

Suitable for patients requiring parenteral nutrition for more than 14 days. Likely candidates include those with:

- inflammatory bowel diseases (e.g. Crohn's disease)
- intestinal atresia
- radiation enteritis
- motility disorders (e.g. scleroderma and chronic idiopathic intestinal pseudo-obstruction syndromes)
- extreme short bowel syndrome.

ADMINISTRATION

Peripheral Line

- Feed is administered into the central venous system using a peripheral vein (refer to Figure 2.7 for access routes). The largest available peripheral vein is accessed using a small cannula or catheter covered with a sterile dressing. A short extension set, to facilitate feeding, is attached to the cannula or catheter.

Central Line Administration

A central venous catheter (CVC) is surgically inserted, aseptically, into the superior vena cava or right atrium (refer to

Figure 2.7 for access routes). The catheter is tunnelled subcutaneously down into the chest to provide a flat surface for applying dressings.

CONTRAINDICATIONS

Absolute Contraindication

• Functioning, usable gut.

Peripheral Parenteral Nutrition

• Insufficient peripheral venous access.
• Unusual feeding regimen that cannot be met by peripheral nutrition.
• Catheter-related infections/complications (although carefully followed aseptic techniques and procedures should prevent this occurring).

Central Line Parenteral Nutrition

• Central line catheter-related infections/complications (although carefully followed aseptic techniques and procedures should prevent this occurring).
• Subcutaneous port device—patients with a needle phobia or fear of injecting through the skin. Refer to 'Feeding tubes' for further information.

FEEDING TUBES (Pennington 1996)

Peripheral

Peripheral feeding is administered using a cannula or catheter device.

Cannula Device

• Administered through any vein.
• <10 cm in length, rigid when held horizontally.
• More suitable for patients requiring peripheral feeding for 1–2 days, as it is less intrusive than long-line feeding catheters.

Catheter Device

- Also known as a 'long line'.
- >10 cm in length, non-rigid when held horizontally.
- Administered subcutaneously into the basilic or cephalic vein.
- Requires patient's arm to be outstretched, so more suitable for immobile or unconscious patients.

Central

There are three main types of single-lumen catheters available, depending on venous access, duration of therapy and patient preference.

Central Venous Catheter (with a Dacron cuff)

- Held in place subcutaneously by fibrous tissue.
- Useful for home parenteral feeding.

Central Venous Catheter (without a Dacron cuff)

- Suitable for feeding over a moderate time, e.g. 2 weeks to 2 months.
- Secured by sutures at exit site; can easily be removed.

Subcutaneous Port

- Small device consisting of an injectable membrane, metal base and catheter limb, secured to the chest wall under the skin.
- Used for home parenteral nutrition.
- Particularly useful when skin sensitivity to dressings is a problem.
- Facilitates greater freedom of activity.

INTRAVENOUS NUTRITION SOLUTIONS
(Adapted from Todorvick & Micklewright 1998)

- Parenteral feeds are contained in aseptic, clear plastic bags (similar to i.v. fluid packaging) ready to hang from a drip stand.

- Parenteral feeding bags contain a mixture of amino acids, glucose, lipids, electrolytes, trace elements and vitamins.

- Pharmacy departments may provide standard 3-litre 'All In One' (AIO) bags containing the above nutrients or specially prepared bags, depending on the individual's nutritional requirements.

- Owing to the osmolarity of standard parenteral feeds and the viability of veins, peripheral feeding often results in a reduced total feed administration.

- A common peripheral line-feeding regimen may consist of 9.4 g nitrogen, 1400–1600 kcal (1000 kcal as lipid), and 3-litre volume.

- Feeds may be covered by a silver bag to prevent sunlight destabilizing fat-soluble vitamins.

- Normally feeding pumps, similar to enteral feeding pumps, will administer the feed.

INITIATING PARENTERAL NUTRITION

Assess:

- nutritional status
- nutritional requirements
- degree of metabolic stress
- expected duration of non-gut access and/or ability to absorb nutrients enterally
- patient's prognosis
- whether a standard or specially prepared feed will be required, e.g. for liver/renal patients or those with a very high/low weight who would be either over- or underfed with a standard feeding bag.

MONITORING (guidelines adapted from Pennington 1996)

- Clinical appearance.
- Daily temperature.

- Daily fluid balance.
- Daily weights.
- Blood glucose, measured 12-hourly for the first 2 days.
- Urea and electrolytes.
- Liver function and haematological tests twice weekly.
- Weekly trace elements and anthropometry (e.g. mid-arm circumference, triceps skin fold thickness and hand grip dynamometry).
- Other blood results as indicated (e.g. vitamin and mineral status).

COMPLICATIONS (Pennington 1996)

Catheter Related
Peripheral Line
- Peripheral vein thrombosis (PVT).

Central Line
- CVC infection or related sepsis.
- Central vein thrombosis.
- Hydrothorax.
- Pneumothorax.
- Haemothorax.
- Air embolisms and catheter embolisms.
- Myocardial perforation.
- Arterial puncture sepsis.

Nutritional and Metabolic Related
- Fluid overload.
- Hyperglycaemia.
- Electrolyte imbalances.
- Symptoms of 'refeeding syndrome' (may occur following severe malnutrition).

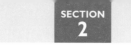
- Micronutrient deficiencies (e.g. in long-term patients receiving home parenteral nutrition).
- Effects of over/underfeeding.

Effects on Other Organ Systems

- Organ systems such as the hepatobiliary system and immune system, and the skeleton, may be affected by parenteral nutrition.

HOME PARENTERAL NUTRITION
(Howard 2000, Wood 1995)

- The main indication for home parenteral feeding is permanent intestinal failure.
- Likely candidates include those with short bowel syndrome, extensive Crohn's disease, radiation to the small intestine, refractory sprue, chronic adhesive obstruction or a diffuse motility gut disorder.
- Delivery of home parenteral feeding requires a multi-disciplinary team approach consisting of physicians, nurses, pharmacists, dietitians, gastroenterologists, surgeons, social workers and pharmaceutical/nutrition company representatives.
- For further information regarding home parenteral nutrition, refer to Howard (2000) and Wood (1995).

REFERENCES

Henry L (1997)
Parenteral nutrition. Professional Nurse 13(1):39–42.

Howard L (2000)
A global perspective of home parenteral and enteral nutrition. Nutrition 16(7–8):625–628.

McAtear CA (ed.) (1999)
Current perspectives on enteral nutrition in adults. British Association for Parenteral and Enteral Nutrition Working Party Report. Maidenhead: BAPEN.

McAtear CA, Wright C (eds) (1996)
Dietetic standards for nutritional support. Birmingham: Parenteral and Enteral Nutrition Group of The British Dietetic Association.

Payne-James J, Grimble G, Silk D (2001)
Artificial nutrition support in clinical practice, 2nd edn. Greenwich: Greenwich Medical Media.

Pennington CR (ed.) (1996)
Current perspectives on parenteral nutrition in adults. British Association for Parenteral and Enteral Nutrition Working Party Report. Maidenhead: BAPEN.

Reilly H (1998)
Enteral feeding: an overview of indications and techniques. Br J Nursing 7(9):510–512, 514–516, 518.

Schneider SM, Pouget I, Staccini P, et al (2000)
Quality of life in long-term home enteral nutrition patients. Clin Nutr 19(1):23–28.

Silk DBA (ed.) (1994)
Organisation of nutritional support in hospitals. British Association for Parenteral and Enteral Nutrition Working Party Report. Maidenhead: BAPEN.

Sizer T (ed.) (1996)
Standards and guidelines for nutritional support of patients in hospital. British Association for Parenteral and Enteral Nutrition Working Party Report. Maidenhead: BAPEN.

Thomas B (ed.) (2001)
Manual of dietetic practice, 3rd edn. Oxford: Blackwell Science.

Todorvick VE, Micklewright A (eds) (1998)
A pocket guide to clinical nutrition, 2nd edn, revised. Birmingham: Parenteral and Enteral Nutrition Group of The British Dietetic Association.

Tortora GJ, Grabowski SR (1999)
Principles of anatomy and physiology, 9th edn. John Wiley.

Whitney EN, Cataldo CB, Rolfes SR (1998)
Understanding normal and clinical nutrition, 5th edn. West/Wadsworth Publishing Company.

Wood S (ed.) (1995)
Home parenteral nutrition: quality criteria for clinical services and the supply of nutrient fluids and equipment. British Association for Parenteral and Enteral Nutrition Working Party Report. Maidenhead: BAPEN.

NUTRITION AND DRUGS

NOTES

- The drugs contained in this section were selected for their effects on nutritional status and nutrition-related diseases. They are intended as a guide only. For a full list of all drugs refer to a current British National Formulary (BNF) or Monthly Index of Medical Specialities (MIMS).

- Drugs are listed by their British Approved Name (BAN), i.e. by their generic, non-proprietary, chemical name. This means that brand-named drugs produced by manufacturers are not listed.

- Recommended International Non-proprietary Names (rINN) for drugs appear, where applicable, in brackets after the BAN, e.g. frusemide (furosemide).

- Owing to the extensive range of vitamin and mineral supplements available, these preparations have not been listed. This information is fully available from a recent edition of a BNF or MIMS.

- Always consult the most recent edition of a BNF or MIMS for a full description of a drug. For further information, consult a clinical pharmacist or drug information line (available in hospitals).

- Unless otherwise stated, the following data have been compiled from the BNF (September 2000).

Table 3.1 Drug–food interactions

Drug	Food type	Effect on drug
ACE inhibitors	Potassium-containing salt substitutes	• May increase serum potassium levels
Acitretin Atovaquone	High-fat meals	• Increase plasma concentrations
Anticoagulants	Foods rich in vitamin K	• Can reduce the effects of warfarin
Azithromycin (not tablet)	Regular meal or snack	• Reduce bioavailability and peak concentrations
Captopril	Regular meal or snack	• Possibly reduces absorption
Ciprofloxacin	Dairy products or enteral tube feeds	• Reduce absorption
Cyclosporin (Ciclosporin)	Food, milk and grapefruit juice	• Increase bioavailability
Didanosine	Regular meal or snack	• Reduces absorption
Digoxin	Bran fibre	• Reduces absorption
Erythromycin stearate	Regular meal or snack	• Reduces absorption
Fluoroquinolones	Iron, magnesium, zinc and calcium supplements	• Reduce absorption
Hydralazine	Food	• Significantly reduces the bioavailability
Isoniazid	Regular meal or snack Foods rich in histamine[a]	• Delays and reduces absorption. May cause a flushing reaction with headache, difficulty in breathing, nausea and tachycardia
Levodopa	High-protein diet	• Competition from amino acids for absorption and transport into the CNS

Table 3.1 Drug–food interactions—continued

Drug	Food type	Effect on drug
Lovastatin	Regular meal	• Increases absorption
MAOIs	Foods rich in tyramine[b]	• May cause a serious hypertensive reaction in some patients
Misoprostol	Regular meal or snack	• Reduces incidence of gastrointestinal adverse effects
Nifedipine	Regular meal or snack Grapefruit juice (concentrated)	• Reduce incidence of adverse effects due to a reduced peak in serum concentrations. Grapefruit juice may cause significant increase in serum concentrations, possibly due to inhibition of nifedipine metabolism
NSAIDs	Regular meal or snack, milk	• Reduce incidence of gastrointestinal effects
Penicillins	Regular meal or snack	• Reduces absorption
Phenytoin	Enteral tube feeding	• Reduces absorption (allow 2 h of rest from feed pre- and post-administration of phenytoin)
Potassium-sparing diuretics	Potassium-containing salt substitutes	• Potential to increase serum potassium level
Rifampicin (rifampin)	Regular meal or snack	• Reduces the absorption of rifampicin from the gut
Sodium clodronate Alendrovic acid Disodium etidronate	Regular meal or snack, iron preparations, calcium supplements, milk and food containing calcium, magnesium and aluminium	• Reduce absorption

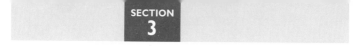

Table 3.1 Drug–food interactions—continued

Drug	Food type	Effect on drug
Sucralfate	Regular meal or snack	• Reduces effect due to binding of protein components in food
Tetracyclines[c]	Regular meal, dairy products, iron	• Reduce absorption due to chelation
Theophylline (regular)	High-carbohydrate, low-protein diet	• Reduces hepatic clearance
Theophylline (sustained release)	Regular meal	• Results in sudden elevation of serum concentrations
Warfarin	Foods high in vitamin K	• Antagonism to the effect of warfarin
Zidovudine	Regular meal or snack	• Reduces absorption

Source: Adapted from Gauthier & Malone (1998).
Abbreviations: MAOIs = monoamine oxidase inhibitors; NSAIDs = non-steroidal anti-inflammatory drugs; CNS = central nervous system.
[a] Histamine-rich foods include cheese and tuna.
[b] Tyramine-rich foods include: cheese, beer, pickled herring, broad bean pods and beef-based hot drinks.
[c] Except doxycycline and minocycline.

Table 3.2 Oral hypoglycaemics (diabetes)

Classification	Action	Side-effects	Drug examples	Comments
Sulphonylureas	• Stimulate the pancreas to release more insulin • Increase the body's sensitivity to insulin	• Generally mild and infrequent • Gastrointestinal disturbances • Headaches	Chlorpropamide[a] Gliclazide[b] Glipizide[b] Tolbutamide[b] Glibenclamide Glimepiride Gliquidone	• Most effective if taken half an hour before food • Can encourage weight gain, so should not be first-line therapy for the overweight • Although there are several sulphonylureas, there is no evidence to suggest any differences in their effects
Biguanides	• Decrease gluconeogenesis • Increase the uptake of glucose by the body tissues	• Initially common and may persist • Nausea/vomiting • Diarrhoea • Risk of lactic acid-osis in patients with renal impairment	Metformin	• Metformin is the only available biguanide • No risk of hypoglycaemia • Most suitable for the overweight (when healthy eating and exercise alone fail to control diabetes)
Other antidiabetics	• Delay the digestion and absorption of starch and sucrose	• Flatulence • Diarrhoea • Abdominal pain	Acarbose	• May be used as first-line therapy or added to other oral hypoglycaemic agents

Table 3.2 Oral hypoglycaemics (diabetes)—continued

Classification	Action	Side-effects	Drug examples	Comments
	• Reduce carbohydrate absorption	• Flatulence • Abdominal distension • Intestinal obstruction	Guar gum	• Must be taken with the first mouthful of a meal • Any glucose taken orally will be absorbed • Cannot cause hypoglycaemia but, if used with other agents, glucose must be used to treat hypoglycaemia (i.e. not sugar) • Also used to relieve symptoms of dumping syndrome • Should be carefully swallowed with water and not taken immediately before going to bed
	• Stimulate insulin release • Rapid onset of action but short duration of activity	• Abdominal pain • Diarrhoea • Constipation • Nausea/vomiting • Hypersensitivity reactions	Repaglinide	• Administer shortly before a meal (dose is omitted if the meal has been missed) • Indicated for NIDDM when healthy eating and exercise fail to adequately control diabetes

Table 3.2 Oral hypoglycaemics (diabetes)—continued

Classification	Action	Side-effects	Drug examples	Comments
	• Increase natural insulin sensitivity	• Weight gain • Headache • Dizziness	Rosiglitazone Dioglitazone	• Can be combined with metformin if metformin alone does not control diabetes • Used in combination with metformin or sulphonylurea where maximum doses of these have failed to control. Contraindicated with insulin

Abbreviation: NIDDM = non-insulin-dependent diabetes mellitus.

a Chlorpropamide has more side-effects than the other sulphonylureas and therefore is no longer recommended.

b Shorter-acting sulphonylureas used in the elderly.

Table 3.3 Insulins[a] (diabetes)

Duration of action	Insulins	Comments
Short-acting	Soluble insulin Insulin aspart Insulin lispro	• Injected subcutaneously (s.c.), relatively rapid onset of action after 30–60 min, then a peak action between 2 and 4 h, and a duration of action of up to 8 h • Aspart and lispro insulins have the advantage of fewer incidences of hypoglycaemia occurring when compared to soluble insulin. They are suitable for those who prefer to inject shortly before or, when necessary, shortly after a meal. Suitable for those prone to prelunch hypoglycaemia and for those who eat late in the evening and are prone to early nocturnal hypoglycaemia
Intermediate/long-acting	Isophane insulin Insulin zinc suspension Protamine zinc insulin Crystalline insulin zinc suspension	• Injected s.c., intermediate and long-acting insulins have an onset of action of approximately 1–2 h, a maximal effect at 4–12 h, and a duration of 16–35 h • Some are given twice daily in conjunction with short-acting (soluble) insulin, and others are given once daily, particularly in elderly patients • Isophane insulin is useful for twice-daily insulin regimens
Mixtures	Biphasic insulin lispro Biphasic isophane insulin	• Mixtures of short- and long-acting insulins

[a] Insulin is the hormone which allows glucose to be utilized by cells for the provision of energy. The duration of action of insulins will differ among patients, and therefore needs to be individually assessed. Insulin requirements may be increased by infection, stress, accidental or surgical trauma and puberty, and during the second and third trimesters of pregnancy. Requirements may be decreased in patients with renal or hepatic impairment and in those with some endocrine disorders, e.g. Addison or coeliac disease. Some patients may only tolerate bovine or porcine insulin and not human insulin. As there are many insulin preparations, refer to a current BNF for more details.

Table 3.4 Anti-diarrhoeal drugs[a]

Presentation	Anti-diarrhoeal drugs	Comments
Acute diarrhoea	Kaolin	• Adsorbent, not recommended for acute diarrhoea
	Ispaghula husk Methylcellulose Sterculia	• Bulk-forming drugs, useful in controlling faecal consistency in ileostomy and colostomy patients. Also used for controlling diarrhoea associated with diverticular disease
	Codeine phosphate Co-phenotrope Loperamide Morphine	• Antimotility drugs. In acute diarrhoea, have a limited role as adjuncts to fluid and electrolyte replacement. Not recommended for acute diarrhoeas in young children. Used for short-term symptomatic relief of acute diarrhoea in adults
Chronic diarrhoea	Mesalazine Olsalazine sodium Sulfasalazine	• Aminosalicylates used for the treatment of mild to moderate ulcerative colitis (UC) and maintenance of remission. Sulfasalazine may be used for treatment of severe UC and Crohn's disease
	Prednisolone	• Corticosteroid used for the treatment of UC and Crohn's disease
	Colestyramine	• Anion exchange resin used for the treatment of diarrhoea associated with Crohn's disease, ileal resection, vagotomy, diabetic vagal neuropathy and radiation
	Sodium cromoglycate	• Cromoglycate, used in the treatment of food allergy (in conjunction with dietary restrictions), asthma, allergic conjunctivitis and allergic rhinitis

[a] The first line of treatment for diarrhoea is to replace lost fluid and electrolytes. Simple gastroenteritis, even when a bacterial cause is suspected, rarely requires drug therapy, since the complaint will usually resolve quickly without such treatment. Systemic bacterial infections (such as *Campylobacter enteritis*, shigellosis or salmonellosis) do, however, require appropriate systemic drug treatment. When a patient has diarrhoea, it is important to exclude any infectious causes (using microbiology laboratory tests) before using antimotility drugs, as this will help to avoid the risk of toxic megacolon.

Table 3.5 Sorbitol[a]-containing drugs (which may cause diarrhoea)

Classification	Sorbitol-containing drugs[b]	Comments
Gastrointestinal	Aluminium- and magnesium-containing antacids	• Several brands containing sorbitol • Sorbitol content ranging from 220 mg/5 ml to 600 mg/5 ml
	Stimulant laxatives	• Two or three brands containing sorbitol • Sorbitol content ranging from 25/200 in 5 ml to 75/1000 in 5 ml
Cardiovascular system	Loop diuretics and potassium-sparing diuretics	• Several brands containing sorbitol • Sorbitol content ranging from 1 mg/5 ml to 100 mg/5 ml
Central nervous system	Drugs used in nausea and vertigo	• Two or three brands containing sorbitol • Sorbitol content ranging from 4 mg/5 ml to 5 mg/5 ml
Nutrition and blood	Oral iron Fluoride Zinc Vitamin D Multivitamin preparations	• Several brands containing sorbitol • Broad range of sorbitol contents

For further information, refer to North West (Liverpool) Drug Information Letter (1998).

[a] Taken in excess, sorbitol may cause diarrhoea. Sorbitol is particularly used in 'sugar-free' formulas such as syrups, liquids, pastilles and suspensions.

[b] Drugs are categorized by BNF classification. Only those directly related to nutrition and dietetics have been selected. Refer to a recent BNF for drug brand names.

Table 3.6 Laxatives[a] (to relieve constipation)

Classification	Laxatives
Bulk-forming	Bran Ispaghula husk Methylcellulose Sterculia
Stimulants	Bisacodyl Danthron (dantron) Docusate sodium Glycerol Senna Sodium picosulphate (sodium picosulfate)
Faecal softeners	Arachis oil Liquid paraffin
Osmotic laxatives	Lactitol Lactulose Macrogols Magnesium salts Phosphates (rectal) Sodium citrate (rectal)

[a] As bowel movement can vary greatly between individuals, constipation may be defined as the passage of hard stools less frequently than the patient's own normal pattern. Before laxatives are prescribed, it is important to establish that the patient is constipated and that the constipation is not secondary to an underlying, undiagnosed complaint. Healthy eating, with sufficient fibre and fluids as well as exercise, is important in preventing constipation (in 'normal', healthy patients). Excessive use of laxatives may lead to hypokalaemia and an atonic non-functioning colon.

Table 3.7 Drugs which may cause constipation

Classification	Drug action
Aluminium-containing antacids, e.g. aluminium hydroxide	• Antacid
Anticholinergics, e.g. tricyclics, phenothiazines	• Drugs used in depression or psychoses and other related disorders
Antihistamines	• Used in the treatment of allergies
Calcium channel blockers, e.g. verapamil	• Used for the treatment of angina, hypertension and arrhythmias
Clonidine	• Centrally acting antihypertensive

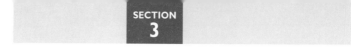

Table 3.7 Drugs which may cause constipation—continued

Classification	Drug action
Diuretics	• Drugs used for the treatment of hypertension and water retention
Iron preparations	• Iron deficiency anaemias
Levodopa, co-beneldopa, co-careldopa	• Drugs used in parkinsonism and related disorders
Monoamine oxidase inhibitors (MAOIs)	• Drugs used for the treatment of phobic and depressed patients
Opiates, e.g. co-proxamol, co-dydramol, morphine	• Opiate-containing analgesics

Table 3.8 Diuretics[a]

Classification	Diuretics
Thiazides (relieve oedema due to heart failure)	Bendrofluazide (bendroflumethiazide) Chlorthalidone (chlortalidone) Cyclopenthiazide Hydrochlorothiazide Indapamide Metolazone Polythiazide Xipamide
Loop (used for pulmonary oedema due to left ventricular failure)	Frusemide (furosemide) Bumetanide Torasemide
Potassium sparing (causes retention of potassium)	Amiloride Triamterene Spironolactone
Potassium sparing with other diuretics	Co-amilozide
Osmotic (used in the treatment of cerebral oedema)	Mannitol
Carbonic anhydrase inhibitors (weak diuretic used in glaucoma)	Acetazolamide

[a] A diuretic is a drug that increases urine volume by promoting the excretion of salts and water from the kidneys. Diuretics are used to reduce oedema due to salt and water retention in disorders of the heart, kidneys or lungs. Some diuretics may be used in conjunction with other drugs to help reduce blood pressure, such as beta-blockers.

Table 3.9 Antiemetics[a]

Antiemetic	Indications
Cinnarizine Cyclizine Dimenhydrinate Meclozine Promethazine hydrochloride Promethazine teoclate	• Vertigo, tinnitus, nausea and vomiting
Chlorpromazine Perphenazine Prochlorperazine Trifluoperazine	• Severe nausea and vomiting due to terminal illness (where other drugs have failed or are not available)
Domperidone	• Acute nausea and vomiting, including that induced by levodopa or bromocriptine, or following chemotherapy or radiotherapy
Metoclopramide	• Nausea and vomiting, particularly in gastrointestinal disorders and treatment with chemotherapy or radiotherapy
Granisetron Ondansetron Tropisetron	• Nausea and vomiting induced by chemotherapy or radiotherapy
Nabilone	• Nausea and vomiting caused by cytotoxic drugs unresponsive to conventional antiemetics (close observation, preferably within an inpatient setting, is required)

[a] Antiemetics relieve symptoms associated with nausea, vomiting and vertigo. They should only be used when the cause of nausea and vomiting is known.

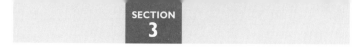

Table 3.10 Appetite stimulants

Appetite stimulants	Comments
Gentian mixture, acid, BP Gentian mixture, alkaline, BP Steroids Alcohol, e.g. sherry	• Causes of reduced appetite are usually multifactorial, e.g. patient suffering from nausea and vomiting, dislike of hospital food, anxiety, stress, unfamiliar hospital environment, drug side-effects, gastrointestinal surgery and so on • Fresh air and gentle exercise (where possible) will help increase appetite. Also encourage patients to have 'favourite' foods/drinks • Avoid encouraging 'favorite' foods/drinks before a patient receives chemotherapy. As patients frequently experience nausea and vomiting following treatment, this may create 'food aversions'

Table 3.11 Dry mouth*[a]* (drug treatment)

Classification	Drugs used for dry mouth	Comments
Local treatment	Artificial saliva sprays Artificial saliva gels Pastilles (formulated for patients suffering from dry mouth)	• Encourage sips of cool drinks, sucking pieces of ice or sugar-free fruit pastilles, chewing gum, sliced citrus fruits and juices
Systemic treatment	Pilocarpine hydrochloride	• For patients with symptoms of xerostomia following radiotherapy for head and neck cancer

[a] Dry mouth (xerostomia) may be caused by drugs with anticholinergic side-effects (e.g. antispasmodics, tricyclic antidepressants and some antipsychotics), by head and neck radiotherapy or by damage to the salivary glands.

Table 3.12 Anti-obesity drugs and appetite suppressants[a]

Classification	Drug	Comments
Anti-obesity drugs (acting on the gastrointestinal tract)	Orlistat	• Reduces the absorption of dietary fat. Licensed for use in conjunction with a reduced energy intake (encouraging a sensible, healthy eating plan) for those with a body mass index of 28–30 and over. Treatment should be started only when a weight loss of 2.5 kg (over 4 consecutive weeks) from diet alone has been achieved. Steatorrhea is a common side-effect
	Methylcellulose	• Most commonly used bulk-forming drug. Reduces dietary intake by producing a feeling of early satiety (but there is no evidence to support this claim). Side-effects include flatulence, abdominal distension and intestinal obstruction
Appetite suppressants (centrally acting)	Phentermine	• Licensed for use as an adjunct to the treatment of selected patients with moderate to severe obesity. Restricted use to 12 weeks or less, so not suitable for the routine management of severe obesity

NB: The appetite suppressants dexfenfluramine and fenfluramine were withdrawn from the market in 1997 following reports of valvular heart disease associated with their use.

[a] Anti-obesity and appetite suppressant drugs are not a sole means of treating obesity (especially in the long term) and are not recommended as the first-line treatment for obesity. If used, they must be used in conjunction with a healthy eating pattern, exercise (where possible) and appropriate lifestyle changes (e.g. cessation of smoking, reducing stress) and for a short period only.

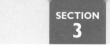

Table 3.13 Lipid-regulating drugs[a]

Classification	Action	Drugs
Anion exchange resins	• Bind bile acids, preventing their reabsorption, promoting hepatic conversion of cholesterol into bile acids. Increases the breakdown of LDL cholesterol	Cholestyramine (colestyramine)
Fibrates	• Main action results in decreased serum TGs. Tend to reduce LDL cholesterol and raise HDL cholesterol	Bezafibrate Ciprofibrate Fenofibrate Gemfibrozil
Ispaghula	• Form of soluble fibre. Likely action is to reduce reabsorption of bile acids. Plasma TGs remain unchanged	Ispaghula
Statins	• Inhibit HMG CoA, involved in cholesterol synthesis, especially in the liver	Atorvastatin Cerivastatin Fluvastatin Pravastatin Simvastatin
Nicotinic acid group	• Lowers both cholesterol and TG concentrations by inhibiting synthesis. Also increases HDL cholesterol	Acipimox Nicotinic acid
Fish oils	• Decrease hepatic VLDL synthesis and increase lipoprotein lipase activity. Reduce plasma TGs in patients with severe hypertriglyceridaemia	Omega-3 marine triglycerides

Abbreviations: LDL = low-density lipoprotein; HDL = high-density lipoprotein; VLDL = very low-density lipoprotein; TG = triglyceride; HMG CoA = 3-hydroxy-3-methylglutaryl coenzyme A.

[a] Appropriate dietary and lifestyle changes must be made before considering any lipid-regulating drug (excluding cases of familial hyperlipidaemia when healthy eating and lifestyle alone cannot control lipid levels adequately). Extensive use of lipid-regulating drugs is not recommended. If lipid-regulating drugs are necessary, they should be used in conjunction with a healthy diet and appropriate lifestyle changes.

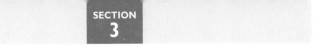
Table 3.14 Irritable bowel syndrome[a] (drugs used to relieve symptoms)

Classification	Drugs
Antispasmodics (to relieve pain)	Atropine Dicycloverine Dicyclomine Hyoscine butylbromide Propantheline
Intestinal smooth muscle relaxants (to relieve pain)	Alverine Mebeverine Peppermint oil

[a] Symptoms of irritable bowel syndrome (IBS) include gastrointestinal pain, constipation and diarrhoea. Stress and psychological factors may aggravate symptoms. Establishing symptoms, current lifestyle (i.e. potential sources of stress-aggravating symptoms) and a dietary assessment will help determine any drug or dietary treatment required.

REFERENCES

British National Formulary (2000)
No. 40. London: The British Medical Association and the Royal Pharmaceutical Society of Great Britain.

Gauthier I, Malone M (1998)
Drug–food interactions in hospitalised patients: methods of prevention. Drug Safety 18(6):383–393.

North West (Liverpool) Drug Information Letter (1998)
Sugar free medicines. No. 113.

NUTRITIONAL SUPPLEMENTS

NOTES

- The nutritional supplements listed in this section reflect those which would be used by dietitians and other health-care professionals for patients in a clinical or community setting.

- Feeds used for paediatrics, metabolic disorders and parenteral nutrition solutions are not included. This information is available from any current British National Formulary (BNF) or Monthly Index of Medical Specialities (MIMS).

- Products are listed by product category, e.g. 'sip feeds', in alphabetical order by product name. Refer to 'Definition of nutritional supplement categories' for more details.

- Nutritional composition is given per total volume or weight of each product. Where more than one volume or weight exists per product, nutritional composition for the lowest measure available is given, unless otherwise stated.

- Slight differences in nutritional composition may occur between different flavours of the same product. In this instance, nutritional composition is given for the predominant similar value among the different flavours. Usually, only flavours such as chocolate raise energy and fat values slightly.

- As a result of a new EC Directive (as from November 2001), for foods used for special medical purposes (FSMP), slight reformulations of some feeds contained in this section may occur.

- Some non-prescription feeds listed in this section may be available on prescription by a named patient system.

- Data were compiled using manufacturers' nutrition services, manufacturers' published product information literature, and the BNF (September 2000). For additional information, refer to the British Dietetic Association (2001).

- All product data are correct, to the best of the author's knowledge, for November 2000. For current and extended information on all nutritional supplements, consult a current BNF, MIMS or manufacturers' nutrition services (refer to Appendix 1 for manufacturers' contact addresses and nutrition help lines).

DEFINITION OF NUTRITIONAL SUPPLEMENT CATEGORIES

Sip Feed

- Product intended to be sipped orally. Most are nutritionally complete, presented as a tetra brick with attached straw.

Enteral Tube Feed

- Any product intended for use as an enteral tube feed, presented in a can, soft pouch/ready to hang, glass or plastic bottle. Most are nutritionally complete. All feeds in this section may also be taken orally but are classed under this category because they are nearly always administered by an enteral feeding tube.

Energy Supplement

- Any product derived from a carbohydrate or fat source (or both) either as a powder or liquid, primarily high in energy only.

Protein Supplement

- Product specifically high in protein, usually in a powder form, but low in most other nutrients.

Thickeners

- Any product in powder form used specifically to thicken food and fluids. Also includes ready-thickened drinks.

Fortified Milk Shakes, Puddings and Soups

- Ready to eat/drink or powder form, fortified with energy, protein and some vitamins and minerals. Most are not nutritionally complete. Some are available on prescription.

PRODUCT INFORMATION KEY

Presentations

Bar	Bar
Box	Box
Can	Can
Combi	Combi block carton
Cup	Cup
DF	Dripac-Flex
Drum	Drum
Gable	Gable top carton

GB	Glass bottle
Jar	Jar
PB	Plastic bottle
Pot	Pot
Sachet	Sachet
SP	Soft pouch/ semi-rigid
Tetra	Tetra brick carton
Tub	Tub

Flavours

ap	Apple
apr	Apricot
asp	Asparagus
ban	Banana
bla	Blackcurrant
but	Butterscotch
cap	Cappuccino
car	Caramel
che	Cherry
chi	Chicken
choc	Chocolate
chocfud	Chocolate fudge brownie
chocmt	Chocolate mint
cit-cola	Citrus-cola
cof	Coffee
cran	Cranberry
d+b	Dandelion and burdock
eg	Egg nog
ff	Fruits of forest Forest fruits
fp	Fruit punch
gr	Grapefruit
honcrun	Honey crunch

lem	Lemon
l+l	Lemon and lime
man	Mandarin
mel	Melon
moc	Mocha
mus	Muesli
mush	Mushroom
n	Neutral
nut	Nut
or	Orange
org	Original
pe	Peach
pear	Pear
pear+che	Pear and cherry
p+o	Peach and orange
p+r	Peach and raspberry
pine	Pineapple
p+l	Potato and leek
ras	Raspberry
r+b	Raspberry and blackcurrant
sf	Summer fruits

str	Strawberry	tom	Tomato
s+r	Strawberry and raspberry	van	Vanilla
		ve	Vegetable
tf	Tropical fruits		Vegetable cream
tof	Toffee		

Manufacturers

Boots	Boots
Fresenius	Fresenius Kabi Ltd
Heinz	H J Heinz Co. Ltd
MJN	Mead Johnson Nutritionals
NCN	Nestlé Clinical Nutrition
Nestlé	Nestlé UK Ltd
Novartis	Novartis Consumer Health, Medical Nutrition Division
NCC	Nutricia Clinical Care, a Division of Nutricia Ltd
Ross	Ross Products, a Division of Abbott Laboratories Ltd
SH	Sutherland Health
SHS	Scientific Hospital Supplies
VF	Vitaflo
UN	Unigreg Ltd

Abbreviations (other)

ACBS	Advisory Committee on Borderline Substances
∗	ACBS approved (i.e. available on prescription)
BCAA	Branched-chain amino acids
g	gram
GI	Gastrointestinal
kcal	kilocalories
kJ	kilojoules
LCT	Long-chain triglycerides
LE	Low in electrolytes
Manufac	Manufacturers
MCT	Medium-chain triglycerides
ml	millilitre
Na	Sodium
Pend	Pending
PKU	Phenylketonuria
Present	Presentation
Volume/wt	Volume/weight

Table 4.1 Sip feeds (milk based)

Product	Manufacturer	Present	Volume/ weight (ml)	ACBS approved	Flavours	Energy kJ (kcal)	Protein (g)	Sodium (mmol)	Potassium (mmol)	Comments
Clinutren ISO	NCN	Cup	200	*	choc, van, cof, str	840 (200)	7.6	3.0	6.7–7.7	Milk-tasting sip feed. 4.18 kJ/ml (1 kcal/ml), gluten-free, nutritionally complete
Clinutren 1.5	NCN	Cup	200	*	van, apr, ban, choc, str	1260 (300)	11.0	7.0	8.8	High-energy milk-tasting sip feed, clinically lactose-free, gluten-free and nutritionally complete. 6.27 kJ/ml (1.5 kcal/ml)
Complan	Heinz	Tetra	230	*	str, van, choc	1050 (250)	8.7	6.0	10.0	Nutritionally complete ready-to-drink sip feed containing skimmed milk and lactose
Ensure Plus	Ross	Tetra	200	*	cof, car, bla, ban, choc, or, van, str, ras, ff, pe, n	1260 (300)	12.5	10.43	10.26	High-energy/low-volume milk-tasting sip feed. 6.27 kJ/ml (1.5 kcal/ml)

Table 4.1 Sip feeds (milk based)—continued

Product	Manufacturer	Present	Volume/ weight (ml)	ACBS approved	Flavours	Energy kJ (kcal)	Protein (g)	Sodium (mmol)	Potassium (mmol)	Comments
Enrich Plus	Ross	Tetra	200	*	van, choc, ras, ban	1285 (305)	12.5	7.39	6.4	High-energy milk-tasting sip feed, with a blend of soluble and insoluble fibre. 1.25 g fibre/100 ml
Entera	Fresenius	Tetra	200	*	van, str, bla, chocmt, but, pine, or, ban, n, ve	1260 (300)	11.3	7–13	9–11.6	High-energy/low-volume milk-tasting sip feed. 6.27 kJ/ml (1.5 kcal/ml)
Entera Fibre Plus	Fresenius	Tetra	200	*	str, van, choc, ban, cap, lem	1260 (300)	11.3	3.5	4.5	High-energy, milk-tasting sip feed containing a mixed fibre blend. 5 g fibre/200 ml tetra
Fortifresh	NCC	Tetra	200	*	ras, bla, man	1298 (300)	12	9.12	10.28	Nutritionally complete, energy-dense, yoghurt-tasting sip feed. 6.27 kJ/ml (1.5 kcal/ml)
Fortimel	NCC	Tetra	200	*	str, ff, van	840 (200)	20	4.34	10.24	High-protein milk-tasting sip feed. Suitable for patients on a sodium restriction. 4.18 kJ/ml (1 kcal/ml)

Table 4.1 Sip feeds (milk based)—continued

Product	Manufacturer	Present	Volume/ weight (ml)	ACBS approved	Flavours	Energy kJ (kcal)	Protein (g)	Sodium (mmol)	Potassium (mmol)	Comments
Fortisip	NCC	Tetra	200	*	ban, or, str, tf, tof, n, van, choc, mush, chi	1270 (300)	12	9.14	10.28	High-energy milk-tasting/low-volume sip feed. 6.27 kJ/ml (1.5 kcal/ml). Chi and mush flavours contain 14.2 mmol sodium per 200 ml
Fortisip Multifibre	NCC	Tetra	200	*	van, str, or, ban, choc	1270 (300)	12	9.14	10.28	High-energy, milk-tasting, sip feed. Enriched with a blend of six fibres. 6.27 kJ/ml (1.5 kcal/ml). 4.5 g fibre per 200 ml
Fresubin	Fresenius	Tetra	200	*	van, nut, pe, choc, moc, bla	840 (200)	7.6	6.6	6.4	Nutritionally complete, milk-tasting sip feed. Suitable for patients on a potassium restriction. 4.18 kJ/ml (1 kcal/ml)

Table 4.1 Sip feeds (milk based)—continued

Product	Manufacturer	Present	Volume/ weight (ml)	ACBS approved	Flavours	Energy kJ (kcal)	Protein (g)	Sodium (mmol)	Potassium (mmol)	Comments
Protenplus	Fresenius	Tetra	200	*	str, van, choc, ff	1050 (250)	20	3.9	3.8	High-protein, high-energy. 5.23 kJ/ml (1.25 kcal/ml) milk-tasting sip feed, rich in vitamins and trace elements and containing fibre (2 g/200 ml tetra)
Resource Shake	Novartis	Combi	175	*	van, choc, str, ban, sf, lem, tof	1278 (304)	8.9	3.0	4.7	A nutritionally balanced, high-energy, ready-to-drink UHT sip feed. 7.1 kJ/ml (1.7 kcal/ml)
Resource Protein Extra	Novartis	Combi	200	Pend	van, choc, sf, apr	1057 (250)	18.8	1.7	2.6	A nutritionally balanced, high-protein, ready-to-drink UHT sip feed. 5.23 kJ/ml (1.25 kcal/ml)

Table 4.1 Sip feeds (milk based)—continued

Product	Manufacturer	Present	Volume/weight (ml)	ACBS approved	Flavours	Energy kJ (kcal)	Protein (g)	Sodium (mmol)	Potassium (mmol)	Comments
Resource Fibre	Novartis	Combi	175	Pend	van, choc, str	1283 (305)	8.9	3.0	4.7	A nutritionally complete ready-to-drink UHT sip feed with added fibre. 7.1 kJ/ml (1.7 kcal/ml)
Sno-Pro	SHS	Tetra	200	*	n	560 (134)	0.44	<6.6	<2.6	Low-protein milk replacer. Also low in phenylalanine (25 mg/unit). Suitable for PKU, inborn errors of metabolism and renal patients. Not a sip feed. Not nutritionally complete

Table 4.2 Sip feeds (fruit flavoured)

Product	Manufacturer	Present	Volume/ weight (ml)	ACBS approved	Flavours	Energy kJ (kcal)	Protein (g)	Sodium (mmol)	Potassium (mmol)	Comments
Clinutren Fruit	NCN	Cup	200	*	or, gr, r+b, pear+che	1040 (250)	8	1.3	2.4	Hydrolysed whey protein. 5.22 kJ/ml (1.25 kcal/ml)
Elemental 028 Extra Liquid	SHS	Tetra	250	*	or+pine, gr, sf	896 (215)	6.2	6.8	6	Amino acid-based fruit-flavoured supplement for patients with severe impairment of the gastrointestinal tract, e.g. short bowel syndrome after intestinal resection, Crohn's disease and intractable malabsorption associated with HIV and bowel fistulas

Table 4.2 Sip feeds (fruit flavoured)—continued

Product	Manufacturer	Present	Volume/ weight (ml)	ACBS approved	Flavours	Energy kJ (kcal)	Protein (g)	Sodium (mmol)	Potassium (mmol)	Comments
Enlive	Ross	Tetra	240	*	or, ap, l+l, pine, str, pe, gr, fp	1275 (300)	9.6	3.04	0.97	Fruit drink-tasting supplement. 5.22 kJ/ml (1.25 kcal/ml)
Fortijuice	NCC	Tetra	200	*	bla, apr, pine, d+b, ff, l+l, p+o	1270 (300)	8	1.3	1.02	Fruit drink-tasting sip feed. 6.27 kJ/ml (1.5 kcal/ml)
Provide Xtra	Fresenius	Tetra	200	*	l+l, ap, bla, mel, che, or+pine, cit-cola	1050 (250)	7.5	2.4	1.2–2.4	High-protein, fruit-tasting, non-milk-based sip feed. Suitable for patients with milk intolerance. 5.22 kJ/ml (1.25 kcal/ml)

Table 4.3 Enteral tube feeds (whole protein)

Product	Manufacturer	Present	Volume/ weight	ACBS approved	Flavours	Energy kJ (kcal)	Protein (g)	Sodium (mmol)	Potassium (mmol)	Comments
Enrich	Ross	Can	250 ml	*	van, choc	1079 (256)	9.4	8.7	9.49	Sip or enteral tube feed. 4.18 kJ/ml (1 kcal/ml), 1.4 g fibre/100 ml (containing non-starch polysaccharides)
Ensure Standard	Ross	Can Tetra	250 ml 200 ml	*	van, choc, cof, eg, chi, nut, asp, mush	1057 (251)	10	9.57	9.49	Sip or enteral tube feed, nutritionally complete. 4.18 kJ/ml (1 kcal/ml)
Ensure Plus	Ross	Can PB PB PB	250 ml 500 ml 1000 ml 1500 ml	* * * *	van	1575 (375)	15.6	13.05	11.6	High-energy/low-volume feed. 6.27 kJ/ml (1.5 kcal/ml)
Fresubin 1000 Complete	Fresenius	SP	1000 ml	*	n	4200 (1000)	55	60	50	Nutritionally complete enteral tube feed containing a mixed fibre blend (2 g fibre/100 ml). 4.18 kJ/ml (1 kcal/ml)
Fresubin 1200 Complete	Fresenius	SP	1500 ml	*	n	5040 (1200)	60	80	72	Nutritionally complete, low-energy, enteral tube feed containing mixed fibre blend

Table 4.3 Enteral tube feeds (whole protein)—continued

Product	Manufacturer	Present	Volume/ weight	ACBS approved	Flavours	Energy kJ (kcal)	Protein (g)	Sodium (mmol)	Potassium (mmol)	Comments
										(2 g fibre/ 100 ml). 3.34 kJ/ml (0.8 kcal/ml)
Fresubin Energy	Fresenius	SP	500 ml 1000 ml	* *	n	3138 (750)	28	21.5	15.9	High-energy/low-volume feed. 6.27 kJ/ml (1.5 kcal/ml)
Fresubin Original	Fresenius	SP SP GB	500 ml 1000 ml 500 ml	* *	n	2100 (500)	19	16.6	16	Nutritionally complete. 4.18 kJ/ml (1 kcal/ml)
Fresubin 750 MCT	Fresenius	SP GB	500 ml 500 ml	*	n	3150 (750)	37.5	26	30	High in protein, energy and MCT. 6.27 kJ/ml (1.5 kcal/ml)
Fresubin Original Fibre	Fresenius	SP SP GB	500 ml 1000 ml 500 ml	* *	n	2100 (500)	19	29	20	Isotonic. 1.5 g fibre/100 ml. 4.18 kJ/ml (1 kcal/ml)
Fresubin Energy Fibre	Fresenius	SP SP	500 ml 1000 ml	*	n	3150 (750)	28	21.7	26.5	Nutritionally complete, high-energy enteral tube feed. 6.27 kJ/ml (1.5 kcal/ml). Contains a mixed fibre blend (2 g fibre/100 ml)
Generaid Plus	SHS	Tub	400 g	*	n	7776 (1852)	44	12	48	Orange-flavoured free amino acid mixture high

Table 4.3 Enteral tube feeds (whole protein)—continued

Product	Manufacturer	Present	Volume/ weight	ACBS approved	Flavours	Energy kJ (kcal)	Protein (g)	Sodium (mmol)	Potassium (mmol)	Comments
										in BCAA. Used in the treatment of hepatic failure for sip or enteral tube feeding
Introlite	Ross	PB	1000 ml		n	2250 (530)	22	39.13	40.26	Low-osmolarity feed with reduced energy. 2.21 kJ/ml (0.53 kcal/ml), and protein, 2.2 g/100 ml, for patients who cannot tolerate full-strength formulas
Isosource Standard	Novartis	SP SP SP	500 ml 1000 ml 1500 ml	*	n	2205 (500)	20.5	15.8	17.3	Standard enteral tube feed. Nutritionally complete. 4.18 kJ/ml (1 kcal/ml)
Isosource Energy	Novartis	SP	500 ml	*	n	5328 (800)	28.5	18.5	17.3	Nutritionally complete, high-energy enteral tube feed. 6.68 kJ/ml (1.6 kcal/ml)
Isosource Fibre	Novartis	SP SP SP	500 ml 1000 ml 1500 ml	*	n	2205 (500)	19.0	15.2	17.3	Standard enteral tube feed with mixed fibres. 4.18 kJ/ml (1 kcal/ml)

Table 4.3 Enteral tube feeds (whole protein)—continued

Product	Manufacturer	Present	Volume/weight	ACBS approved	Flavours	Energy kJ (kcal)	Protein (g)	Sodium (mmol)	Potassium (mmol)	Comments
Jevity	Ross	PB PB PB	500 ml 1000 ml 1500 ml	* * *	n	2205 (525)	20	19.5	20.1	4.18 kJ/ml (1 kcal/ml) feed, 1.1 g fibre/100 ml, enriched with fructo oligosaccharide (FOS)
Jevity Plus	Ross	PB PB PB	500 ml 1000 ml 1500 ml		n	2520 (600)	28	29.35	3.75	Higher-energy fibre feed with FOS. 5 kJ/ml (1.2 kcal/ml), 1.2 g fibre/100 ml
Modulen IBD	NCN	Can	400 g	*	n	8160 (2000)	72	29.2	62.4	Whole protein disease-specific formula—Crohn's disease, contains MCT. Gluten- and lactose-free. 20.9 kJ/g (5 kcal/g)
Nepro	Ross	Can	237 ml	*	van	1988 (475)	16.6	8.7	6.41	For renal patients on dialysis. Low-electrolyte sip or enteral tube feed. 8.36 kJ/ml (2 kcal/ml)
Novasource GI Control	Novartis	SP GB SP	500 ml 500 ml 1500 ml	*	n	2205 (500)	20.5	15.2	17.3	Enteral tube feed with soluble fibre. 4.18 kJ/ml (1 kcal/ml)

Table 4.3 Enteral tube feeds (whole protein)—continued

Product	Manufacturer	Present	Volume/weight	ACBS approved	Flavours	Energy kJ (kcal)	Protein (g)	Sodium (mmol)	Potassium (mmol)	Comments
Novasource GI Forte	Novartis	SP	500 ml	Pend	n	3155 (750)	30	18.5	17.3	High-energy, enteral tube feed with soluble fibre. 6.27 kJ/ml (1.5 kcal/ml)
Nutrison concentrated LE	NCC	SP GB	500 ml 500 ml		n	4200 (1000)	37.5	21.5	19	Energy-dense feed for patients requiring restricted fluid and electrolyte intakes. 8.36 kJ/ml (2 kcal/ml), 7.5 g protein/100 ml
Nutrison Energy	NCC	GB SP SP SP	500 ml 500 ml 1000 ml 1500 ml	* * * *	n	3150 (750)	30	29	25.7	High-energy, low-volume feed. 6.27 kJ/ml (1.5 kcal/ml)
Nutrison Multi Fibre	NCC	GB SP SP SP	500 ml 500 ml 1000 ml 1500 ml	* * * *	n	2100 (500)	20	21.75	19.2	4.18 kJ/ml (1 kcal/ml), 1.5 g fibre/100 ml
Nutrison Low Protein Mineral	NCC	GB SP	500 ml 500 ml		n	4200 (1000)	20	21.5	19	Low-protein, energy-dense feed. For use in renal/liver patients. 8.36 kJ/ml (2 kcal/ml)

Table 4.3 Enteral tube feeds (whole protein)—continued

Product	Manufacturer	Present	Volume/ weight	ACBS approved	Flavours	Energy kJ (kcal)	Protein (g)	Sodium (mmol)	Potassium (mmol)	Comments
Nutrison Low Na	NCC	GB SP	500 ml 1000 ml		n	2100 (500)	20	5.5	17.5	Low in sodium (1.1 mmol/100 ml). 4.18 kJ/ml (1 kcal/ml)
Nutrison Pre	NCC	GB SP	500 ml 1000 ml		n	1046 (250)	10	10.85	9.75	Hypotonic, half-strength feed for patients who cannot tolerate full-strength feeds or require extra fluid. 2.09 kJ/ml (0.5 kcal/ml)
Nutrison Soya	NCC	GB SP	500 ml 1000 ml	* *	n	2092 (500)	20	21.75	19.2	Isotonic, milk-free . feed 4.18 kJ/ml (1 kcal/ml)
Nutrison Standard	NCC	GB SP SP SP	500 ml 500 ml 1000 ml 1500 ml	* * * *	n	2100 (500)	20	21.75	19.2	Isotonic feed. 4.18 kJ/ml (1 kcal/ml)
Osmolite	Ross	Can PB PB PB	250 ml 500 ml 1000 ml 1500 ml	* * * *	n	1060 (252)	10	9.77	9.48	Isotonic feed. 4.18 kJ/ml (1 kcal/ml)

Table 4.3 Enteral tube feeds (whole protein)—continued

Product	Manufacturer	Present	Volume/ weight	ACBS approved	Flavours	Energy kJ (kcal)	Protein (g)	Sodium (mmol)	Potassium (mmol)	Comments
Osmolite Plus	Ross	PB PB PB	500 ml 1000 ml 1500 ml		n	2540 (605)	28	28.25	23.2	Higher in energy than standard enteral tube feed, providing 5 kJ/ml (1.2 kcal/ml)
Oxepa	Ross	PB	500 ml	*	n	3165 (750)	31.25	28.5	25.15	Contains omega-3 fatty acids, specially formulated for patients with acute lung injury and compromised respiratory function. 6.27 kJ/ml (1.5 kcal/ml)
Pulmocare	Ross	Can PB PB	250 ml 500 ml 1000 ml		van	1577 (377)	15.75	14.12	12.54	Nutritional values per 250-ml can. High-fat, low-carbohydrate feed, designed for patients with compromised respiratory function. 6.27 kJ/ml (1.5 kcal/ml)
Reconvan	Fresenius	SP	500 ml		n	2100 (500)	27.5	30	26.5	Nutritionally complete, high-glutamine enteral tube feed enriched with arginine and omega-3 fatty acids

Table 4.3 Enteral tube feeds (whole protein)—continued

Product	Manufacturer	Present	Volume/weight	ACBS approved	Flavours	Energy kJ (kcal)	Protein (g)	Sodium (mmol)	Potassium (mmol)	Comments
Sondalis	NCN	DF	500 ml 1000 ml	* *	n	2100 (500)	39	26	30	Isotonic milk-free, containing MTCs. 4.18 kJ/ml (1 kcal/ml)
Sondalis 1.5	NCN	DF	500 ml 1000 ml	* *	n	3200 (750)	56	48	44	High-energy/low-volume enteral tube feed with MTCs. 6.27 kJ/ml (1.5 kcal/ml)
Sondalis Fibre	NCN	DF	500 ml 1000 ml	*	n	2100 (500)	38	26	30	Fibre-enriched standard feed. Multisource MTCs. 4.18 kJ/ml (1 kcal/ml)
Sondalis Hp	NCN	DF	500 ml		n	2800 (670)	34	17	19	High-protein, gluten-free, clinically lactose-free. 6.7 g protein/100 ml
Suplena	Ross	Can	237 ml	*	n	1994 (476)	7.1	8.26	6.82	For patients with protein, fluid and electrolyte restrictions. Sip or enteral tube feed. 4.18 kJ/ml (1 kcal/ml)
Two Cal HN	Ross	Can	237 ml	*	n	2010 (479)	19.8	13.48	14.72	For catabolic patients following severe trauma. 8.36 kJ/d (2 kcal/ml)

Table 4.4 Enteral tube feeds (elemental and semi-elemental)

Product	Manufacturer	Present	Volume/ weight	ACBS approved	Flavours	Energy kJ (kcal)	Protein (g)	Sodium (mmol)	Potassium (mmol)	Comments
AlitraQ	Ross	Sachet	76 g		van	1277 (302)	15.8	13.04	9.23	Nutritional values per 300 ml (reconstituted as directed). Glutamine-enriched, low-fat, enteral tube feed to meet the needs of critically ill patients. Contains MCT oil. 4.18 kJ/ml (1 kcal/ml)
Dialamine	SHS	Tub	200 g	*	or	3060 (720)	50	<0.8	<0.6	Orange-flavoured amino acid mixture, designed to give optimum essential amino acid intake. For oral or enteral tube feeding. May be used for advanced chronic renal failure. Not nutritionally complete
Elemental 028	SHS	Sachet	100 g	*	or, n	1614 (382)	10	10.8	11.9	High osmolarity, hypoallergenic, low fat. Amino acid based

Table 4.4 Enteral tube feeds (elemental and semi-elemental)—continued

Product	Manufacturer	Present	Volume/ weight	ACBS approved	Flavours	Energy kJ (kcal)	Protein (g)	Sodium (mmol)	Potassium (mmol)	Comments
E028 Extra liquid	SHS	Sachet	100 g	*	or, n	1793 (427)	12.5	13.3	11.9	Hypoallergenic, elemental, and increased nitrogen, fat, energy, glutamine and arginine
Emsogen	SHS	Sachet	100 g	*	or, n	1839 (438)	12.5	13	11.9	Most fat as MCT (83%)
Hepatamine	SHS	Tub	60 g		or	918 (216)	15	0.24	0.18	For use in hepatic failure. Supplement added to enteral tube feed. Contains BCAAs
Nutrison MCT	NCC	GB SP	500 ml 1000 ml	* *	n	2100 (500)	25	21.75	19.2	MCT enteral tube feed, gluten-free. For patients with short bowel syndrome and fat malabsorption
Pepdite 1+	SHS	Can	400 g	*	n	1844 (439)	13.8	9.1	13.2	Nutritional values per 100 g powder. Sip or enteral tube feed. Milk protein-free, gluten-free, lactose-free, sucrose-free, and fructose-free. Used for malabsorption-related diseases, e.g. bowel fistulae

Table 4.4 Enteral tube feeds (elemental and semi-elemental)—continued

Product	Manufacturer	Present	Volume/weight	ACBS approved	Flavours	Energy kJ (kcal)	Protein (g)	Sodium (mmol)	Potassium (mmol)	Comments
Peptamen	NCN	Cup Can DF DF	200 ml 375 ml 500 ml 1000 ml		van n n n	840 (200)	8.0	5.2	5.6	Nutritional values per 200-ml cup. Whey based, average peptide length 8 amino acid units. 70% fat MCT, unflavoured (neutral) hypotonic, vanilla isotonic. 4.18 kJ/ml (1 kcal/ml)
Peptamen Flavoured	NCN	Cup Sachet	200 ml 18 × 3 g	* *	van, ban, str, cof, choc, I+I n	840 (200)	8	5.2	5.6	Per 200-ml van flavour. Added to Peptamen for flavour (cup presentation available in van flavour only)
Pepti (liquid)	NCC	GB SP SP	500 ml 500 ml 1000 ml	* * *	n	2100 (500)	20	21.75	19.2	Semi-elemental, low fat. 4.18 kJ/ml (1 kcal/ml)
Pepti (powder)	NCC	Sachet	126 g	*		2073 (489)	18	10.2	18.1	Semi-elemental, low fat. Reconstituted for patients with inflammatory bowel disease and malabsorption

Table 4.4 Enteral tube feeds (elemental and semi-elemental)—continued

Product	Manufacturer	Present	Volume/ weight	ACBS approved	Flavours	Energy kJ (kcal)	Protein (g)	Sodium (mmol)	Potassium (mmol)	Comments
Perative	Ross	Can	237 ml	*	n	1308 (310)	15.8	10.87	10.51	Nutritional values per 237-ml can. Semi-elemental. 5.43 kJ/ml (1.3 kcal/ml)
		PB	500 ml	*						
		PB	1000 ml	*						
Reabilan	NCN	Can	375 ml	*	n	1575 (375)	12	11	13	Semi-elemental. 4.18 kJ/ml (1 kcal/ml)
		SP	500 ml	*						
Survimed OPD	Fresenius	GB	500 ml	*	n	2100 (500)	22.5	29	20	Low fat, semi-elemental, average peptide chain length 2.7 amino acids. 4.18 kJ/ml (1 kcal/ml)
		SP	500 ml							

Table 4.5 Fortified milk shakes (powders)

Product	Manufacturer	Present	Volume/ weight	ACBS approved	Flavours	Energy kJ (kcal)	Protein (g)	Sodium (mmol)	Potassium (mmol)	Comments
Build Up	NCN	Sachet Box	38 g × 4 266 g		l+l, str, van, choc, ban, org	1350 (270)	15.6	12.9	18.2	Nutritional values per 38-g sachet made up with 200 ml whole milk
Calshake Powder	Fresenius	Sachet	87–90 g	*	ban, str, choc, van	2502 (598)	12	9.7	11.2	Nutritional values per one sachet (87–90 g) made up with 240 ml whole milk. High-energy powdered supplement
Complan	Heinz	Sachet Box	57 g × 4 450 g		ban, choc, org, p+r, str, van	1057 (251)	8.8	5.7	10.8	Nutritional values per 57-g sachet made up with 200 ml water. Can also be reconstituted with milk
Recovery	Boots	Sachet Box	55 g × 4 500 g		org, str, choc	1459 (348)	18	13	19.3	Nutritional values per 55-g sachet made up with 200 ml whole milk
Scandi-shake	SHS	Sachet	85 g	*	van, str, choc	2505 (598)	11.7	10.9	26.0	Nutritional values per 85-g sachet made up with 240 ml whole milk. High-energy milkshake

Table 4.6 Fortified puddings

Product	Manufacturer	Present	Volume/ weight	ACBS approved	Flavours	Energy kJ (kcal)	Protein (g)	Sodium (mmol)	Potassium (mmol)	Comments
Cinutren Dessert	NCN	Pot	125 g	*	pe, van, choc, car	650 (160)	12	8.1	7.9	Semi-solid, high-protein, milk-tasting pudding for patients with dysphagia
Formance	Ross	Pot	113 g	*	van, choc, but	711 (170)	4	5.83	4.6	Semi-solid nutritional supplement
Forti-pudding	NCC	Tub	125 g	*	choc, cof, van, ff	857 (201)	12.5	4.0	6.75	Semi-solid, high-protein, milk-tasting pudding-for patients with dysphagia
Maxisorb	SHS	Sachets	30 g	*	choc, str, van	579 (138)	12	1.8	4.1	High-protein dessert mix
Resource Energy Dessert	Novartis	Pot	125 g	Pend	van, choc, car	841 (200)	6	2.2	4.2	Semi-solid, high-protein, milk-tasting pudding for the management of disease-related malnutrition and dysphagia

Table 4.7 Fortified soups

Product	Manufacturer	Present	Volume/ weight	ACBS approved	Flavours	Energy kJ (kcal)	Protein (g)	Sodium (mmol)	Potassium (mmol)	Comments
Build Up	NCN	Sachets	49–51g		chi, p+l, tom, ve	885–915 (210–220)	8–10.2	30.1–34.4	6.5–9.5	Nutritional values per 49–51 g sachet made up with 200 ml water. High in sodium, negligible fibre. Not nutritionally complete
Complan	Heinz	Sachets	57 g × 4		chi, ve	1033 (245)	8.8	32.2	6.9	Nutritional values per 57-g sachet made up with 200 ml water. High in sodium
Vita-savoury	VF	Cup Sachet	33 g 50 g	* *	chi; p+l, mush	870 (210)	4	15.7	0.86	Nutritional values per 33-g cup made up with 70 ml water. Energy-dense savoury supplement, reconstituted with water. 8.36 kJ/ml (2 kcal/ml) when reconstituted

Table 4.8 Energy supplements

Product	Manufacturer	Present	Volume/ weight	ACBS approved	Flavours	Energy kJ (kcal)	Comments
Calogen	SHS	GB	250 ml 1000 ml	* *	but, str, n	4625 (1125)	LCT fat emulsion. 18.81 kJ/ml (4.5 kcal/ml)
Caloreen	NCN	Can	500 g	*	n	8159 (1950)	Glucose polymer. 16.3 kJ/ml (3.9 kcal/g)
Calsip	Fresenius	Tetra	200 ml	*	ap, pine, n	1680 (400)	High-energy, low-volume liquid carbohydrate supplement. 8.36 kJ/ml (2 kcal/ml)
Duobar	SHS	Bar	100 g	*	str, van	2692 (648)	Fat and carbohydrate in solid form, protein-free
Duocal Liquid	SHS	GB GB	250 ml 1000 ml	* *	n	1653 (395)	Fat and glucose polymer, protein-free. 6.68 kJ/ml (1.6 kcal/ml)
Duocal Super Soluble	SHS	Tub	400 g	*	n	8244 (1968)	Fat and glucose polymer, protein-free
Ensure Bar	Ross	Bar	38 g	*	chocfud, honcrun	587 (139)	Nutritionally complete. Suitable for patients on fluid restriction. 6.5 g protein, 3.26 mmol sodium and 4.72 mmol potassium per 38-g bar
Liquigen	SHS	GB GB	250 ml 1000 ml	* *		4625 (1125)	MCT fat emulsion. 16.72 kJ/ml (4 kcal/ml)
Maxijul Liquid	SHS	Tetra	200 ml	*	bla, l+l, or, n	1700 (400)	Glucose polymer liquid. 8.36 kJ/ml (2 kcal/ml)
Maxijul LE	SHS	Can Tub	200 g 2 kg	* *	n	3230 (760)	Glucose polymer, low in electrolytes. 15.88 kJ/ml (3.8 kcal/ml)

Table 4.8 Energy supplements—continued

Product	Manufacturer	Present	Volume/ weight	ACBS approved	Flavours	Energy kJ (kcal)	Comments
Maxijul Super Soluble	SHS	Sachet Tub Drum Drum	132 g 200 g 2.5 kg 25 kg	* * * *	n	2132 (502)	Glucose polymer. 15.88 kJ/ml (3.8 kcal/ml)
MCT Duocal	SHS	Tub	400 g	*	n	8168 (1944)	Mostly MCT fat and glucose polymer (83%). 20.9 kJ/g (5 kcal/g)
MCT Oil	SHS	GB	500 ml	*	n	17 575 (4275)	MCT oil, 35.53 kJ/ml (8.5 kcal/ml)
MCT Oil	MJN	GB	950 ml	*	n	30 685 (7334)	MCT oil, 32.26 kJ/ml (7.72 kcal/ml)
Polycal Powder	NCC	Tub	400 g	*	n	6460 (1520)	Glucose polymer powder, 15.88 kJ/g (3.8 kcal/g)
Polycal Liquid	NCC	GB	200 ml	*	apr, ap, bla, lem, or, n	2100 (494)	Glucose polymer solution, 10.45 kJ/ml (2.5 kcal/ml)
Polycose	Ross	Tub	350 g	*	n	5264 (1316)	Glucose polymer, 15.88 kJ/ml (3.8 kcal/ml)
QuickCal	VF	Sachet	13 g	*	n	422 (101)	Fat and carbohydrate powder supplement. 32.6 kJ/g (7.8 kcal/g)
Vitajoule	VF	Sachet Tub Tub Tub	130 g 500 g 2.5 kg 25 kg		n	2093 (494)	Glucose polymer, 15.88 kJ/ml (3.8 kcal/ml)

Table 4.9 Protein supplements

Product	Manufacturer	Present	Volume/ weight	ACBS approved	Flavours	Protein (g)	Comments
Casilan 90	Heinz	Box	250 g	*	n	225	0.9 g protein/g
Forceval Protein	UG	Sachet Sachet	30 g 36 g	* *	str, van, choc, n	16.5	Calcium caseinate with 25 vitamins and minerals. 0.55 g protein/g
Maxipro Super Soluble HBV	SHS	Tub Tub	200 g 1 kg	* *	n	160	Whey protein powder concentrate supplemented with amino acids. For use in hypoproteinaemia. 0.8 g protein/g
Pro-Cal	VF	Sachet Tub Tub Tub	15 g 510 g 1.5 kg 12.5 kg	* * * *	n	13.5	Nutritional values per 100 g powder. Protein, fat and carbohydrate food enricher
Promod	Ross	Tin	275 g	*	n	206	Concentrated source of high-quality protein (whey and lecithin). 0.75 g protein/g
Protifar	NCC	Tub	225 g	*	n	199	Concentrated milk powder protein. 0.8 g protein/g
Vitapro	VF	Tub Tub	250 g 1 kg	* *	n	187	Milk protein. 0.75 g protein/g

Table 4.10 Thickeners

Product	Manufacturer	Present	Volume/weight	ACBS approved	Flavours	Comments
Nestargel	Nestlé	Tub	125 g	*	n	Carob seed flour and calcium lactate. A natural thickening agent indicated for use in the dietary management of infantile or adult vomiting, including nausea and vomiting during pregnancy
Nutilis	NCC	Tub	225 g		n	Modified maize starch
Resource Thicken Up	Novartis	Tub	225 g	*	n	Modified food starch indicated for patients requiring thickening of liquid or food
Thick and Easy	Fresenius	Tub	225 g	*	n	Modified maize starch and maltodextrin
		Tub	4.5 kg	*		
Thick and Easy Thickened Juices	Fresenius	PB	1350 ml	*	ap, or, cran	A pre-thickened fruit juice drink mixed to a honey consistency
Thixo-D	SH	Tub	375 g	*	n	Modified maize starch
Thixo-D Drink Mixes	SH	Tub	560 g		ban, choc, or, str	High-energy, thickened drinks
Thixo-D Cal-Free	SH	Tub	30 g		n	Xanthan gum, energy-free thickener
Vitaquick	VF	Tub	100 g	*	n	Modified maize starch
		Tub	300 g	*		
		Tub	1 kg	*		
		Tub	6 kg	*		

REFERENCES

British Dietetic Association (2001)
Advisor enteral tube and sip feeding chart: summarised data for the nutritional composition and presentation of enteral tube and sip feeds. Birmingham: The British Dietetic Association.

British National Formulary (2000)
No. 40. London: The British Medical Association and the Royal Pharmaceutical Society of Great Britain.

GENERAL NUTRITIONAL AND MEDICAL DATA

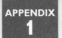

NOTES

- Appendix 1 covers a range of general nutritional and medical data which student dietitians on clinical placement and other health professionals may find useful.

- Always use reference ranges, e.g. for clinical blood bio-chemistry, as set by your hospital.

- Medical abbreviations and shorthand will vary from different hospitals; so use those as set by your hospital.

- Refer to a current British National Formulary (BNF) or Monthly Index of Medical Specialities (MIMS) for up-to-date information on nutrition manufacturers' contact details.

Table A1.1 Useful conversion factors

Parameter	Conversion factor			
Weights and measures	$1 oz = 28.35 g = \sim 1–2$ tablespoons			
	$16 oz = 453.6 g = 1 lb = 0.45 kg$			
	$5 g = \sim 1$ teaspoon			
	$1 stone = 14 lbs = 6.35 kg$			
	$1 kg = 2.2 lbs = 1000 g$			
	$1 pt = 568 ml$			
	$1 l = 1000 ml = 1.76 pt$			
	$1 g = 1 ml = 1000 mg$			
	$1 ft = 0.31 m = 30.48 cm$			
Energy from macronutrients	$1 kcal = 4.184 kJ$			
	$1 g Fat = 9 kcal = 38 kJ$			
	$1 g Alcohol = 7 kcal = 36 kJ$			
	$1 g Protein = 4 kcal = 17 kJ$			
	$1 g Carbohydrate = 3.75 kcal = 17 kJ$			
Protein equivalent	$1 g AA = 0.833 g$ Protein			
Nitrogen equivalent	$1 g Nitrogen = 6.25 g$ Protein			
Sodium (Na)	$1 mmol Na^+ = 23 mg Na^+ = 58.5 mg NaCl$			
	$1 g Na = 43.5 mmol Na^+ = 2.5 g NaCl$			
	$1 g NaCl = 17.1 mmol Na^+ = 393 mg Na$			
	$1 g NaHCO_3 + 12 mmol Na^+ = 327 mg Na$			
	$1 g MSG = 5.2 mmol Na^+ = 120 mg Na$			
	$1 l$ normal saline $= 150 mmol Na^+ = 3450 mg Na$			
Potassium (k)	$1 mmol K^+ = 39 mg K = 74.6 mg KCl$			
	$1 g K^+ = 25.6 mmol K^+ = 1.9 g KCl$			
Vitamins	Vitamin D $1 \mu g = 40 IU$			
	Vitamin E $1 mg = 1 IU$			
mg → mmol	$\dfrac{mg}{\text{atomic weight}}$			
mmol → mg	$mg = mmol \times$ atomic weight			
Atomic weights	Sodium	23.0	Potassium	39.0
	Calcium	40.0	Chloride	40.0
	Chloride	35.4	Magnesium	24.3
	Phosphorus	31.0	Sulphur	32.0

Abbreviations:

g = grams	l = litre	mg = milligram	ml = millilitre
IU = international units	mmol = millimole	μg = microgram	kJ = kilojules
	lb = pound	kg = kilogram	
kcal = kilocalories	oz = ounce	pt = pint	

Table A1.2 Clinical blood biochemistry reference ranges

Parameter/ units	Normal ranges	Comments
Sodium mmol/l	130–147	Hyponatraemia (low sodium) may indicate overhydration (i.e. excessive fluid intake) or an insufficient dietary sodium intake. Diuretics may cause low sodium levels (as increased urine output increases sodium output). Hypernatraemia (high sodium) usually indicates dehydration or is indicative of reduced renal function
Potassium mmol/l	3.3–5.5	Often affected in renal failure or with diuretic treatment. Can partly reflect hydration status. In renal patients, aim to keep levels <6. Both hyper- and hypokalaemia can lead to cardiac dysfunction
Urea mmol/l	1.7–8.3 (20–30 normal for renal patients)	Raised urea and sodium levels can indicate some renal impairment or dehydration. Low levels can indicate overhydration
Creatinine μmol/l	Males 60–125 Females 55–106	Raised levels can indicate renal impairment
Creatinine clearance ml/min	Males 95–140 Females 85–125	Used to measure glomerular filtration rate (indicative of renal function). Raised levels can also indicate muscle protein degradation and negative nitrogen balance
Phosphate mmol/l	0.8–1.6	Raised levels can indicate impaired renal function. Aim to keep levels <2.0 in renal patients. If low can affect adenosine triphosphate (ATP) synthesis (mainly seen in critically ill patients)

Table A1.2 Clinical blood biochemistry reference ranges—continued

Parameter/ units	Normal ranges	Comments
Albumin g/l	36–53	Poor short-term indicator of protein malnutrition, since trauma, diseased states (such as liver and renal disease) and level of hydration can all affect level. Low albumin reduces oncotic pressure, increasing risk of ascities/oedema
Total protein g/l	66–87	Low levels may indicate protein malnutrition
Corrected calcium (Ca) (for albumin) mmol/l	2.20–2.26	Corrected for albumin of 42 mmol/l. Albumin carries Ca around the body, so a low albumin may result in a low calcium level. Equation to calculate corrected Ca when albumin is <40 = measured calcium mmol/l + $$\frac{(40 - \text{serum albumin})}{40}$$ Use corrected Ca or obtain ionized Ca levels at all times
Fasting plasma glucose concentration mmol/l	3.5–5.5	Fasting levels $\geqslant 7.0$ indicates Diabetes. Refer to p. 131 for further details on diabetes diagnostic criteria
Glycosylated haemoglobin (HbA1c)%	6.5–7.5 <8 8.1–9.6 >10	• Excellent Shows an average • Good blood glucose • Suboptimal control over past • Poor 6–8 weeks
Haemoglobin (Hb) g/dl	M 13.0–18.0 F 11.5–16.5	More direct measure of iron deficiency than haematocrit readings. Raised levels caused by dehydration/polycythemia.

Table A1.2   Clinical blood biochemistry reference ranges—continued

Parameter/ units	Normal ranges	Comments
		Decreased levels with haemorrhage/anaemia/protein–energy malnutrition. In renal patients, erythropoeitin injections start when levels are <8.0
Iron (Fe) μmol/l	M 14–31 F 11–29	Raised values associated with iron overload/haemolytic disorders/acute liver damage. Low levels occur with iron deficiency anaemia/nephrosis infections
Total cholesterol mmol/l	3.4–5.2	A combination of lifestyle, genetics and diet will affect serum cholesterol levels. Serum cholesterol levels should be measured alongside other serum lipid parameters such as HDL, LDL and TGs for a more accurate lipid profile. Elevation of serum cholesterol levels, up to approximately 1 month, is common following a heart attack
High-density lipoprotein (HDL) mmol/l	M 0.94–1.44 F 1.16–1.66	Transports excess cholesterol from cells to the liver for excretion in bile. High levels are beneficial and inversely related to heart disease
Low-density lipoprotein (LDL) mmol/l	<4	Transports cholesterol from the liver to peripheral tissues. 60% of total cholesterol is found in LDL. LDL cholesterol is most closely associated with heart disease
Triglycerides (TG) mmol/l	0.8–1.9	Raised levels are associated with heart disease. Dietary TGs are hydrolysed in the intestines and

1

Table A1.2 Clinical blood biochemistry reference ranges—continued

Parameter/ units	Normal ranges	Comments
		formed into micelles with bile salts and cholesterol
Vitamins		Unlikely to routinely screen for
A μmol/l	0.7–1.7	all serum vitamin levels in
B_1 nmol/l	>40	hospital, since expensive and
B_2 nmol/l	Total <85.0 Free <21.3	requires specialized equipment
B_6 nmol/l	>178	
B_{12} ng/l	160–925	Vitamin B_{12} injections may be
Ascorbate μmol/l	34–68	necessary for patients who have had a total gastrectomy, due to
D nmol/l	24–111	loss of intrinsic factor
E μmol/l	10.2–39.0	
pH	7.35–7.45	>7.45 = alkalosis <7.35 = acidosis
Bicarbonate mmol/l	22–32	Often altered in lung, kidney and liver disease. Affects acid–base balance
Chloride mmol/l	95–107	Useful in determining the cause of acidosis
Bilirubin μmol/l	0–19	Increased levels indicate jaundice
Gamma GT u/l	M <50 F <40	
Alanine amino-transferase u/l	7–40	
Alkaline phosphatase ium/u/l	M 60–306 F 30–130	
Creatinine kinase (CK) u/l	M <195 F <170	Main cardiac enzyme measurement. Raised levels may indicate infarcted myocardial tissue, but may also reflect other damaged body tissue

Reference ranges based on The Royal London and The Royal Hallamshire, Sheffield, Hospital Figures.
Interpretation of parameters, Hope et al (1998).

DIABETES DIAGNOSTIC CRITERIA (Alberti 1998)

Diabetes symptoms (i.e. polyuria, polydipsia and unexplained weight loss) plus:

- a random venous plasma glucose concentration $\geqslant 11.1$ mmol/l, or

- a fasting plasma glucose concentration $\geqslant 7.0$ mmol/l (whole blood $\geqslant 6.1$ mmol/l), or

- 2-h plasma glucose concentration $\geqslant 11.1$ mmol/l 2 h after 75 g anhydrous glucose in an oral glucose tolerance test (OGTT).

NB: A diagnosis should not be based on a single glucose determination when no symptoms are present. Allow at least one additional confirmatory glucose test result on another day (either fasting, from a random sample or from a 2-h post-glucose load). If the fasting or random values are not diagnostic, the 2-h value should be used.

MEDICAL ABBREVIATIONS

A

AA	amino acid	AIDS	Acquired immune deficiency syndrome
AAA	abdominal aortic aneurysm	AKA	above-knee amputation
AB	antibiotics	ALS	amyotrophic lateral sclerosis
abdo	abdominal		
ACBS	Advisory Committee on Borderline Substances	Amb	ambulant, ambulatory/ ambulance
ACEvits	vitamins A, C and E	A&E	Accident and Emergency
AD	Alzheimer's disease	ALL	acute lymphocytic leukaemia
ADH	antidiuretic hormone		
AF	atrial fibrillation	al	albumin
AFB	acid-fast bacilli	AML	acute myelogenous or myeloid leukaemia
A/G	albumin/globulin ratio		
AI	aortic insufficiency/ incompetence	AN	anorexia nervosa or antenatal
AID	artificial insemination (donor)	ANF	antinuclear factor
		ADL	activities of daily living

AP	anterioposterior	ASD	arterial septal defect
A–R	apical–radical (pulse)	ASHD	arteriosclerotic heart
ARDS	acute respiratory distress		disease
	syndrome	ATN	acute tubular necrosis
ARF	acute renal failure	AV	arteriovenous/
AS	alimentary system		atrioventricular
ASAP	as soon as possible	A+W	alive and well
ASCVD	arteriosclerotic	AXR	abdominal X-ray
	cardiovascular disease		

B

BaE	barium enema	BNO	bowels not open
BBB	bundle branch block	BOR	bowels open regularly
BCAA	branched-chain amino acid	BP	blood pressure
BID	brought in dead	BS	blood sugar/bowel
BKA	below-knee amputation		sounds/breath sounds
BM	blood sugar/glucose levels	BT	brain/breast tumour
	or bowel movement	BMI	body mass index
BMTU	Bone Marrow Transplant	BMR	basal metabolic rate
	Unit	BUN	blood urea nitrogen
BMTX	Bone Marrow transplant	Bx	biopsy
BNF	British National		
	Formulary		

C

c̄	with	CDH	children's day hospital
c̲	without	C/E	Church of England
Ca	carcinoma, calcium	CEA	carcinoembryonic anti-
CABG	coronary artery bypass		body
	graft	CF	cystic fibrosis
CAL	chronic airways limitation	CHD	coronary heart disease
CAPD	continuous ambulatory	CHF	congestive heart failure
	peritoneal dialysis	CHO	carbohydrate
CAT	computer-assisted tomog-	CL	clubbing
	raphy	CLD	chronic liver disease
Cath.	catholic or catheter	CMH	community and mental
CBC	complete blood count		health
CCF	chronic cardiac failure/	CML	chronic myeloid
	congestive cardiac failure		leukaemia
CCPD	continuous cyclical	CMV	cytomegalovirus
	peritoneal dialysis	CNS	central nervous system
CCU	coronary care unit	C/N	charge nurse
CDC	Centers for Disease	CRG	cardiac rehabilitation group
	Control	CRP	C-reactive protein

C/O	complains of	C+S	culture and sensitivity
C/S	Church of Scotland	CSF	cerebrospinal fluid
COAD	chronic obstructive airway disease	CSU	catheter specimen of urine
		C/T	continue treatment
COLD	Chronic obstructive lung disease	CT	computed tomography
		CVA	cerebrovascular accident/ costovertebral angle
COPD	chronic obstructive pulmonary disease	CVD	cardiovascular disease
CPK	creatinine phosphokinase	CVP	central venous pressure
CPR	cardiopulmonary resuscitation	CVS	cardiovascular system
		Cx	cervix
CRF	chronic renal failure	CXR	chest X-ray
CS	cardiovascular sysem	Cy	cyanosis

D

D	diagnosis	DOA	dead on arrival
D&C	dilation and curettage	DOE	dyspnoea on exertion
DC	discharge, discontinue, decrease	DTs	delirium tremens
		DTR	deep tendon reflexes
DD	differential diagnosis	DU	duodenal ulcer
DIC	disseminated intra vascular coagulation	DUB	dysfunctional uterine bleeding
DM	diabetes mellitus	D+V	diarrhoea and vomiting
DN	district nurse	DVT	deep vein thrombosis
DNS	diabetes nurse specialist	D/W	discussed with
DNA	did not attend (outpatients)	DXT	deep X-ray therapy

E

EAA	essential amino acid	EMG	electromyography
ECG	electrocardiogram	EMIT	enzyme immune assay
EDC	expected date of confinement	ENG	electronystagmogram
		EOM	extracellular movement
EDD	expected date of delivery	ERCP	endoscopic retrograde cholangiopancreatography
ECT	electroconvulsive therapy		
EEG	electroencephalogram	ESR	erythrocyte sedimentation rate
EFA	essential fatty acids		
ENT	ears, nose and throat	EXP	expansion

F

FA	folic acid	FBS	fasting blood sugar
FB	finger breadth/foreign body	FEV	forced expiratory volume in 1 second
FBC	full blood count	FH	family history

FLP	fasting lipid profile	FUO	fever of unknown origin
FROM	full range of movement	Fx, #	fracture, latter symbol
FTND	full term, normal delivery		also used as dose of
FTT	failure to thrive		radiation

G

g	gauge	GS	genital system
gast	gastrostomy	GSD	glycogen storage disease
GB	gall bladder	GT	gamma glutamyl
GC	gonococci		transferase
GCS	Glasgow coma scale	GTT	glucose tolerance test
GFR	glomerular filtration rate	GUM	genitourinary medicine
GI, GIT	gastrointestinal tract	gyn	gynaecology

H

Hb, Hgb	haemoglobin	HEENT	head, eyes, ears, nose and
HbAlc	glycosylated		throat
	haemoglobin	H & P	history and physical
HCVD	hypertensive cardiovascu-	HPC	history of present
	lar disease		condition
HD	haemodialysis	HO	house officer
HDL	high-density lipoprotein	HPI	history of present illness
HDU	high-dependency unit	HTVD	hypertensive vascular
HIV	human immunodeficiency		disease
	virus	HV	health visitor, home visit

I

IBD	irritable bowel disease	I+O	intake and output
ICM	intracostal margin	IP	intraperitoneal
ICS	intercostal space	IPD	intermittent peritoneal
ICP	intracranial pressure		dialysis
ICU	intensive care unit	ISQ	in status quo
IDDM	insulin-dependent diabetes	i.v.	intravenous
	mellitus	IVC	intravenous
I&D	incision and drainage		cholecystogram
IHD	intermittent haemodialysis/	IVP	intravenous pyelogram
	ischaemic heart disease		

J

J	jaundice	JVP	jugular venous pressure

K

KO	keep open	KVO	keep vein open
KS	Kaposi's sarcoma		

L

L	lymphadenopathy	LLL	left lower lobe (lung) or left lower lid (eye)
L	left		
LAT	lateral	LLQ	left lower quadrant (abdomen)
LBBB	left bundle branch block		
		LMP	last menstrual period
LBW	low birth-weight	LOW	loss of weight
LCFA	long-chain fatty acid	LP	lumbar puncture
LCT	long-chain triglyceride	LSB	long-stay bed (geriatric)
LDL	low-density lipoprotein	LTX	liver transplant
LD	lethal dose	LUQ	left upper quadrant (abdomen)
LE	lupus erythematosus		
LFT	liver function test	LVF	left ventricular failure
LIH	left inguinal hernia	LVH	left ventricular hypertrophy
LKS	liver, kidney, spleen		

M

M	murmur	MI	myocardial infarction, mitral incompetence, mitral insufficiency
MCFA	medium-chain fatty acids		
MCH	mean corpuscular haemoglobin		
		MMA	methyl malonic acidemia
MCHC	mean corpuscular haemo-globin concentration	MND	motor neuron disease
		MRI	magnetic resonance imaging
MCT	medium-chain triglyceride		
MCL	midclavicular line	MS	multiple sclerosis, mitral stenosis
MCV	mean corpuscular volume		
METS	metastases	MSU	midstream urine
MF	myocardial fibrosis, mycoses fungoides	MSUD	maple syrup urine disease
		MTA	mid-thigh amputation

N

N	normal	#NOF	fractured neck of femur
NAD	nothing abnormal detected, no acute distress	NPN	non-protein nitrogen
		NS	nervous system (1–12 cranial nerves; T tone; P power; C coordination; S sensitive)
NBM	nil by mouth		
NEC	necrotizing enterocolitis		
NHL	non-Hodgkin lymphoma		
NIDDM	non-insulin dependent diabetes mellitus	NSR	normal sinus rhythm
		N+V	nausea and vomiting

O

OA	on admission, osteoarthritis	Ob-Gyn	obstetrics and gynaecology
		O/D	overdose
OB	occult blood	OE	on examination

OOB	out of bed	OT	old tuberculin, occupational therapy
OPA	outpatient appointment		
OR	operating room	OU	both eyes
Orthop-	orthopnea	O	absent, e.g. OBS = no bowel sounds
OS	left eye		

P

PA	propionic acidemia, posterio-anterior, pernicious anaemia	PN	percussion note
		PND	paroxysmal nocturnal dyspnoea
PARA	number of pregnancies	PNET	primitive neuroectodermal tumour
PAT	paroxysmal atrial tachycardia		
PBC	primary biliary cirrhosis	PND	post-nasal drip
PBI	protein-bound iodine	PO	per os (by mouth)
PC	present condition, after meals	POD	paracetamol overdose
		POLY	polymorphonuclear leukocytes
PCP	*Pneumocystis carini* pneumonia	PPD	purified protein derivative (of tuberculin), packs per day
PCN	penicillin		
PCV	packed cell volume	PPH	postpartum haemorrhage
PE	physical examination, pulmonary embolism		
		PPN	peripheral parenteral nutrition
PEC	pneumoencephalogram		
PEG	percutaneous endoscopic gastrostomy	PPT	partial prothrombin time
PERRLA	pupils equal, round, reactive to light and accommodation	PR	plantar response, per rectum
		prn	when required
		pt	patient
PET	pre-eclamptic toxaemia	PT	prothrombin time, physiotherapy
PF	peak flow		
PID	prolapsed intervertebral disc, pelvic inflammatory disease	PTA	prior to admission
		PTR	prothrombin ratio
PKU	phenylketonuria	PTT	partial thromboplastin time
PM	post mortem		
PMB	postmenopausal bleeding	PU	peptic ulcer
		PUO	pyrexia of unknown origin
PMH	past medical history		
PMI	point of maximum impulse	PV	per vagina
		PVC	premature ventricular contraction
PMN	polymorphonuclear leukocytes		

R

R	right	RLL	right lower lobe
RA	rheumatoid arthritis, right auricle/atrium	RLQ	right lower quandrant
		RQ	respiratory quotient
RBBB	right bundle branch block	R/O	rule out
RBC	red blood count, red blood cell	ROS	review of symptoms
		RR	recovery room
RBS	random blood sugar	RS	respiratory system
RF	rheumatoid factor or respiratory failure	RSV	respiratory syncytial virus
		RTA	road traffic accident
RFT	respiratory function tests	RTX	renal transplant
		RUQ	right upper quadrant
RHD	rheumatic heart disease	RVH	right ventricular hypertrophy
RLE	right lower extremity		

S

S	symptoms	SCID	severe combined immune deficiency
S1	first heart sound		
S2	second heart sound	SDH	subdural haematoma
SA	sinoatrial	SED	slow efficient dialysis
SAH	subarachnoid haemorrhage	SH	social history
SALT	speech and language therapist	SHO	senior house officer
		s.l.	sublingual
SB	seen by	SLE	systemic lupus erythematosus
SBE	subacute bacterial endocarditis		
		SOA	swelling of ankle
s.c.	subcutaneous	SOB	shortness of breath or stools for occult blood
sc	subclavian		
SC	sclerosing cholangitis	SOS	swelling of sacrum
SCC	squamous cell carcinoma or spinal cord compression	SR	sedimentation rate
		SRD	state-registered dietitian
		STD	sexually transmitted disease
SCFA	short-chain fatty acids		

T

T&A	tonsillectomy and adenoidectomy	TIA	transient ischaemic attack
TAH	total abdominal hysterectomy	TIBC	total iron-binding capacity
		TKVO	to keep vein open
TB	tuberculosis	TLC	total lung capacity or tender loving care
TBA	to be arranged (outpatients)		
TCA	to come again (outpatients)	TM	tympanic membrane
TCC	transitional cell carcinoma	TOF	trachaeo-oesophageal fistula
TG	triglyceride		

TPI	*Treponema pallidum* immobilization	TTA	to take away (medications and equipment)
TPN	total parenteral nutrition	TURP	transurethral resection of prostate
TPR	temperature/pulse/ respiration	TX	treatment, therapy
TSH	thyroid-stimulating hormone		

U

UA	uric acid, urinalysis	URTI	upper respiratory tract infection
UC	ulcerative colitis		
U+E	urea and elctrolytes	US	urinary system, ultrasound
UGI	upper GI series	UTI	urinary tract infection

V

| v | very | VLBW | very low birthweight |
| Vanc | vancomycin | | |

W

| WCC | white cell count | W/E | weekend |

X

| xs | excess | | |

Z

| ZF | zimmer frame | | |

Main sources: Entwistle (1998), Hope et al (1998) and Thomas (2001).

Table A1.3 Medical shorthand

×/7	× days or × times a week	2nd	second
×/52	× weeks	2c	to see
×/12	× months	♀	female
∴	therefore	♂	male
→	resulting in	+ +	an excess of
1°	primary	×	times
2°	secondary	×, ✓	dislikes, likes
+ve	positive	2222 or 55	resuscitation
−ve	negative	#	fracture
↑	increase	<	less than
↓	decrease	>	greater than
↔	stable	△	diagnosis
1st	first	◇	abdomen

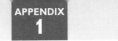

Table A1.4 Pharmaceutical abbreviations

Abbreviation	Dose	Abbreviation	Dose
o.d.	once a day	p.r.n.	when required
b.d.	twice a day	a.c.	before food
t.d.s.	three times a day	p.c.	afer food
q.d.s.	four times a day	o.m.	in the morning
q.q.h.	every 4 hours	o.n.	at night

Table A1.5 Chemical elements and symbols

A		H		P	
Ag	Silver	H	Hydrogen	P	Phosphorus
Al	Aluminium	He	Helium	Pb	Lead
As	Arsenic	Hg	Mercury	Pt	Platinum
Au	Gold				
		I		**R**	
B		I	Iodine	Ra	Radium
B	Boron				
Ba	Barium	**K**		**S**	
Be	Beryllium	K	Potassium	S	Sulphur
Bi	Bismuth			Se	Selenium
Br	Bromine	**L**		Si	Silicon
		Li	Lithium	Sn	Tin
C				Sr	Strontium
C	Carbon	**M**			
Ca	Calcium	Mg	Magnesium	**T**	
Cd	Cadmium	Mn	Manganese	Ti	Titanium
Cl	Chlorine	Mo	Molybdenum	Tl	Thallium
Co	Cobalt			Tu	Tungsten
Cr	Chromium	**N**			
Cu	Copper	N	Nitrogen	**U**	
		Na	Sodium	U	Uranium
F		Ni	Nickel		
F	Fluorine			**V**	
Fe	Iron	**O**		V	Vanadium
		O	Oxygen		
G				**Z**	
Ga	Gallium			Zn	Zinc

Table A1.6 Amino acids in humans

Essential amino acids[a]	Non-essential amino amids	Branched-chain amino acids
Isoleucine	Alanine	Leucine
Leucine	Arginine	Isoleucine
Lysine	Aspartic acid	Valine
Methionine	Cystine	
Phenylalanine	Glutamic acid	
Valine	Glycine	
Threonine	Histidine	
Tryptophan	Hydroxyproline	
	Proline	
	Serine	
	Tyrosine	
	Ornithine	

[a] Essential amino acids cannot be synthesized by humans, so they have to be obtained through dietary sources.

Table A1.7 Nutrition and dietetic internet sites

Internet site	Internet address
Anthropometry Information	www.nutritionclassroom.com
The British Dietetic Association	www.bda.uk.com
Bristish Association for Parenteral and Enteral Nutrition (BAPEN)	www.bapen.org.uk
The American Dietetic Association	www.eatright.org/
Coeliac Society	www.coeliac.co.uk
British Diabetic Association	www.diabetes.org.uk
Dietetics Online	www.dietetics.com/
The 'Virtual' Nutrition Centre	www-sci.lib.uci.edu/~martindale/
Nutrition Society	www.nutsoc.org.uk/
Food and Nutrition Information Centre	www.nalusda.gov/fnic/
World Health Organization	www.who.ch/
Hospital Web	neuro-www.mgh.harvard.edu/ hospitalweb.shtml
The Visible Human Project	www.nlm.nih.gov/research/ visible/visible_human.html
Pharmaceutical Information Network	pharminfo.com/pin_hp.html
The British Medical Journal	www.bmj.com/bmj/

For further information refer to Anagnostelis & Welsh (2000).

Table A1.8 UK manufacturers' addresses for nutritional supplements

Manufacturer	Address
Baxter Healthcare Ltd	Caxton Way, Thetford, Norfolk IP24 3SE
(Mead Johnson) Bristol-Myers Squibb Pharmaceuticals Ltd	141-149 Staines Rd, Hounslow, Middlesex TW3 3JB T: (020) 8572 7422
Everfresh Natural Foods	Gatehouse Close, Aylesbury, Bucks HP19 3DE T: (01296) 425333
Fresenius Kabi Ltd	6/8 Christleton Court, Stuart Rd, Manor Park, Runcorn, Cheshire WA7 1ST T: (01928) 594257
General Dietary Ltd	PO Box 38, Kingston Upon Thames Surrey KT2 7YP T: (020) 8336 2323
Gluten Free Foods Ltd	270 Centennial Park, Centennial Avenue, Elstree, Borehamwood, Herts WD6 3SS T: (020) 8953 4444
Heinz H J Co Ltd	Stockley Park, Uxbridge UB11 1HZ T: (020) 8573 7757
Hypoguard (UK) Ltd	Dock Lane, Melton, Woodbridge, Suffolk IP12 1PE T: (01394) 387333
Jacobs Bakery Ltd	PO Box 1, Long Lane, Liverpool L9 7BQ T: (0151) 525 3661
(Boots) Knoll Ltd	9 Castle Quay, Castle Boulevard Nottingham NG7 1FW T: (0115) 912 5000
Milupa Ltd	Whitehorse Business Park, Trowbridge, Wilts BA14 0XB
Monmouth Pharmaceutical Ltd	20 Nugent Rd, The Surrey Research Park, Guildford, Surrey GU2 5AF T: (01483) 565299

Table A1.8 UK manufacturer's addresses for nutritional supplements—continued

Manufacturer	Address
Nestlé Clinical Nutrition	St George's House, Park Lane, Croydon, Surrey CR9 1NR T: (020) 8667 5130
Nestlé UK Ltd	St Georges House, Croydon, Surrey CR9 1NR T: (020) 8686 3333
Norgine Ltd	Chaplin House, Moorhall Rd, Harefield, Middlesex UB9 6NS T: (01895) 826600
Nova Nordisk Pharmaceuticals Ltd	Broadfield Park, Brighton Rd, Pease Pottage, Crawley, West Sussex RH11 9RT T: (01293) 613555
Novartis Nutrition UK Ltd	Wimblehurst Rd, Horsham, West Sussex RH12 5AB T: (01403) 210211
Nutricia Clinical Care Ltd	White Horse Business Park, Trowbridge, Wiltshire BA14 0XQ T: (01225) 711677
Nutrition Point Ltd	13 Taurus Park, Westbrook, Warrington, Cheshire WA5 5ZT T: (07041) 544044
Panpharma Ltd	Panpharma House, Repton Place, White Lion Rd, Little Chalfont, Amersham, Bucks HP7 9LP T: (01494) 766866
Pharmacia and Upjohn Ltd	Milton Keynes Energy Park Davey Avenue, Knowlhill, Milton Keynes, Bucks MK5 8PH T: (01908) 661101
Robinson Healthcare	Waterside, Walton, Chesterfield Derbyshire S40 1YF T: (01246) 220022

Table A1.8 UK manufacturer's addresses for nutritional supplements—continued

Manufacturer	Address
Roche Products Ltd	40 Broadwater Rd, Welwyn Garden City, Herts AL7 3AY T: (01707) 366000
Ross Products Division	Abbott Laboratories Ltd, Abbott House, Nolden Road, Maidenhead, Berkshire SL6 4XE T: (0800) 252882
Salt and Sons Ltd	Saltair House, Lord St, Nechells, Birmingham, B7 4DS T: (0121) 359 5123
Scientific Hospital Supplies (UK) Ltd	100 Wavertree Boulevard, Wavertree Technology Park, Liverpool L7 9PT T: (0151) 228 8161
Smithkline Beecham Consumer	11 Stoke Poges Lane, Slough, Berkshire SL1 3NW T: (01753) 533433
Sunderland Health Ltd	Unit 5, Rivermead, Pipers Way Thatcham, Berks RG13 4TP T: (01635) 874488
Unigreg Ltd	Enterprise House, 181/191 Garth Rd, Morden, Surrey SM4 4LL T: (0181) 330 1421 Unigreg Nutrition Helpline Freephone 0800 373 698 Email: Admin@Unigreg.co.uk
Vitaflow Ltd	11 Century Building, Brunswick Business Park, Liverpool L3 4BL T: (0151) 709 9020
Wyeth Laboratories	Huntercombe Lane South Maidenhead, Berks SL6 0PH T: (01628) 604377

Source: Adapted from BNF (2000).

Table A1.9 Nutrition and dietetic addresses

Society	Address
British Association of Parenteral and Enteral Nutrition (BAPEN)	PO Box 922, Maidenhead, Berkshire SL6 4SH T: (01628) 644162
British Diabetic Association	10 Queen Anne St, London W1G 9LH T: (020) 7323 1531 F: (020) 7637 3644 Email: info@diabetes.org.uk
British Dietetic Association	7th Floor, Elizabeth House 22 Suffolk St, Queensway, Birmingham B1 1LS T: (0121) 616 4900 F: (0121) 616 4901 Email: info@bda.uk.com
Coeliac Society	PO Box 220, High Wycombe, Bucks HP11 2HY T: (01494) 437278 F: (01494) 474349
Council for Professions Supplementary to Medicine	Park House, 184 Kennington Park Rd, London SE11 4BU T: (020) 7582 0866 F: (020) 7820 9684
Eating Disorders Assoication	Wensum House, 1st Floor, 103 Prince of Wales Road, Norwich NR1 1DN T: (01603) 619090 F: (01603) 664915 Email: eda@netcom.co.uk
The Vegan Society	7 Battle Rd, St Leonards-on-Sea, East Sussex TN37 7AA T: (0142) 442 7393 F: (0142) 471 7064 Email: info@vegansociety.com
The Vegetarian Society	Parkdale, Durham Rd, Altrincham, Cheshire WA14 4QG T: (0161) 925 2000 F: (0161) 926 9182 Email: info@vegsoc.org

APPENDIX
1

REFERENCES

Alberti KG (1998)
Definition, diagnosis and classification of diabetes mellitus and its complications. Part 1: diagnosis and classification of diabetes mellitus provisional report of a WHO consultation. *Diabet Med* 15(7):539–553.

Anagnostelis B, Welsh S (2000)
Finding and using health and medical information on the internet. Aslib.

British National Formulary (2000)
No. 40. London: The British Medical Association and The Royal Pharmaceutical Society of Great Britain.

Entwistle IR (1998)
Exacta medica: reference tables and data for the medical and nursing professions, 2nd edn. Edinburgh: Churchill Livingston.

Hope RA, Longmore JM, McManus SK, et al (1998)
Oxford handbook of clinical medicine, 4th edn. Oxford: Oxford University Press.

Thomas B (ed.) (2001)
Manual of dietetic practice, 3rd edn. Oxford: Blackwell Scientific Publications.

DIETETIC CLINICAL PLACEMENT

NOTES

- Appendix 2 aims to cover significant areas associated with student dietetic clinical placement. However, it is not intended as a comprehensive list of all clinical placement training areas.

- Divided into six parts, this section covers: dietetic clinical placement, hospital catering systems, the medical team, medical records, dietetic referral procedures and dietetic case studies.

- Although these areas have been frequently separated, they are interlinked.

- For a content and timescale impression of a clinical placement timetable, refer to Table A2.1.

- Each student's experience of clinical placement will differ according to the individual, base trainer and hospital. However, by the end of clinical placement, all students should have the same level of dietetic clinical competence.

- For convenience, documents produced by The British Dietetic Association (BDA), referenced in this section, have been abbreviated to 'BDA'.

- In all cases, follow the procedures and practices of your base trainer.

Dietetic Clinical Placement

- While the 'old' system is gradually being phased out, there are currently two clinical placement systems in operation: the 'old' system, consisting of one clinical training block; and the new system, consisting of three separate clinical training blocks.

- This section describes the structure of clinical training for both systems.

- Not all universities and base trainers will immediately transfer to the new system. From year 2000, there will be a period of approximately 8 years until the old system is completely phased out. Both systems will therefore be in operation until this time.

- The term 'base trainer' refers to the nutrition and dietetic departments training the student dietitians on their clinical placements (approved by The Dietitians' Board for the clinical training of dietetic students).

Hospital Catering Systems

- Usually, during the beginning of clinical placement, you will have time to become familiar with your hospital's catering system. This may involve spending time in the catering department and/or reading relevant information.

The Medical Team

- Members of the multidisciplinary team (e.g. professions allied to medicine, PAM) have not been discussed in any detail here. During ward times you will become familiar with different PAM staff and may shadow and/or attend presentations held by PAM members.

Medical Records

- Throughout the medical notes, doctors will use medical abbreviations and shorthand such as those used in this section; to familiarize yourself with them, refer to Appendix 1.

Dietetic Referral Procedures

- Refer to Appendix 3 for diet history and dietetic patient interviewing information.

Dietetic Case Studies

- Case studies will normally be undertaken once you have become competent at understanding and retrieving patient medical and dietetic information. Main case studies may be commenced approximately halfway through placement (but this will vary among different students and base trainer practices).

Table A2.1 Example of a previous and new clinical placement timetable

	Previous placement structure	New placement structure	
Week	Activity[a]	Placement/Year	Activity
1	Department induction. Familiarization with hospital layout, office and catering procedures/work	A Year 1 or 2 4 weeks	Awareness Can take place in a hospital, catering, community or GP setting. Introduction to placement setting, e.g. in a ward environment: familiarity with ward surroundings and staff. Observing: dietitian interviewing patients, ward and catering procedures
2	Catering management/Diet bay		
3	Ward week. Shadow nurses on specific ward. Familiarization with staff gradings and ward procedures		
4–8	Shadow dietitian(s) for general dietetic in/outpatients, including obese, diabetic, malnourished and enterally tube-fed patients Begin to interview patients, take diet histories, document in medical/dietetic and nurse's records (supervised). Assignment of individual tasks, e.g. computer dietary analyses, 'mini case studies'	B[b] Year 3 and/or 4 12 weeks	Building Can take place in any of the above settings. Learn 'core' dietetics (e.g. malnourished, overweight, diabetic, lipidlowering and enterally tube-fed patients). May do small verbal case study presentation(s). Possibly do 1 week of ward work at the end, regularly reporting back to appropriate dietitian (e.g. on a general medical ward)
9–13	Shadow senior dietitians, e.g. renal, community, paediatric, liver and diabetes dietitians. Begin main case study		

Table A2.1 Example of a previous and new clinical placement timetable—continued

Previous placement structure		New placement structure	
Week	Activity[a]	Placement/Year	Activity
14–17	3-week holiday (1 week of this would normally be taken at another time)	C[b] Year 3 and/or 4 12 weeks	Consolidation Working in a hospital, clinical setting. Consolidation of existing knowledge and practical application of 'core' dietetics. Overview of speciality dietetics. May do small verbal case study presentation(s). Main, written case study completed. 2 weeks of ward work at the end, reporting regularly back to responsible dietitian
18–22	Complementary placement, consolidate existing knowledge of general dietetic patients. Expand on area(s) of interest		
23–26	Shadow specialist dietitian(s). Study days, e.g. specialist dietetic departments in surrounding areas, talks, lectures		
27–31	4 weeks of ward and outpatient management, unaccompanied, but regularly reporting back to responsible dietitian(s). Main case study completed. Final appraisal and assessment		

[a] This timetable is based on the author's own experiences as a dietetic student on clinical placement, so always use the timetable devised by your base and complementary trainer.

[b] Blocks B and C should be done with no shorter period of time than 4 weeks between them.

Dietetic Clinical Placement

INTRODUCTION

- The aim of clinical placement is to train the student to a competent level expected of a newly qualified dietitian.

- Patients commonly seen include: malnourished, diabetic, obese, lipidlowering and enterally tube-fed patients.

- Clinical placement also provides an overview of various dietetic specialities, e.g. paediatrics, burns, renal.

- Students will undertake one main patient case study during their clinical placement (refer to p. 175 for more details).

- For an account of a student's experience during clinical placement, refer to Byrne (2000).

PREVIOUS PLACEMENT SYSTEM

- 6-week catering placement (usually completed in year 1 or year 2).

- 31-week clinical training block (24 weeks at a base training hospital, 4 weeks at a complementary hospital and 3 weeks' holiday). Refer to Table A2.1 for an example of a clinical placement timetable.

- Prior to placement, you will receive, from your academic institute, information concerning all base training hospitals, to help you choose your base trainer. Complementary placement is usually chosen during the early weeks of clinical placement.

- Approximately 2–3 months prior to placement, your base trainer will send you information regarding your hospital and accommodation. Not all base trainers provide hospital accommodation, so establish this with your base trainer before you commence placement.

- Some base trainers may schedule your 3 weeks' holiday in your timetable before you commence placement. If you have already booked a holiday, ensure that you inform your base trainer of this in good time.

- Half a day per week private study time should be allocated within your timetable.

- Each supervising dietitian will assess and discuss your progress with you, so that your strengths, skills or knowledge that require more work, and interests, can be developed.

- Identify your base trainer student mentor, so that you can discuss any queries or problems you may have during placement.

- Approximately halfway through clinical placement, a course tutor from your academic institute will normally visit you and your base trainer, to review your progress. You may also have a formal half-time assessment interview by your base trainer.

- During the last 4 weeks of clinical placement, you will be responsible for various ward, and outpatient clinic(s), unsupervised, but reporting back regularly to the appropriate dietitian(s).

- For further information, refer to Dietitians' Board/BDA (1991) and BDA (2000a).

NEW PLACEMENT SYSTEM

- The new placement system will incorporate three practical placements over the course of study.

- Placement A will be for 4 weeks in year 1 or year 2. Placements B and C will be for 12 weeks each in year 3 and/or year 4 (refer to Table A2.1).

- The previous 6-week catering placement, usually done in year 1 or year 2, will no longer exist. Students will, however, acquire an appreciation of catering management and of the relationships between dietetic and catering services during the three new placements.

- Each base trainer will use the learning outcomes in the pre-registration, education and training manual (Dietitians' Board 2000). This is a standard document used by all base trainers dealing with students on the new placement system. Students will need to demonstrate competence and complete the aims and learning outcomes from this document before they can proceed to the next placement.

- Students will keep and maintain their own portfolio of evidence, e.g. as a reflective diary or as evidence of work experience completed. This may be signed, on completion of each task, by the student and supervisor.

- For further information, refer to Dietitians' Board (2000) and BDA (2000a).

Hospital Catering Systems

- Hospital menus commonly follow a 2- or 3-week cycle.

- External catering systems now operate in many hospitals; that is, food is prepared off-site by a catering contractor, commonly using 'cook–chill' methods.

- Some hospital catering departments will have a diet bay or diet cook(s) who can prepare special menus (such as adding protein and energy supplements or artificial sweeteners to foods).

- Meals are usually served at ward level, using a hot-plate 'bulk' system or an individually trayed and portion-controlled system.

- Patients may receive breakfast at around 8.00 a.m., lunch at 12.00 p.m. and an evening meal at 6.00 p.m., although this will vary greatly among different hospitals and wards.

- Generally speaking, patient mealtimes are not good times to see a patient (unless you wish to observe meal distribution at ward level or a patient's dietary intake). Try mid-morning or mid-afternoon instead.

- Depending on budget holders, nutritional supplements may be stored at ward level, within the catering departments, or within the pharmacy and/or dietetic department.

- The patient's charter states that no patient should have to order more than 1 day's meals in advance and that ethnic menus should be available.

The Medical Team

DOCTORS

House Officers (HOs)

• Newly qualified doctors (called 'pre-registration doctors') begin work on the wards as their first appointment. HOs work for a specific consultant and are supervised by a senior house officer (SHO) for 1 year before becoming fully registered. Six months of this time will be spent on medical wards, and 6 months on surgical wards.

• For new patients, HOs will prepare the patient's investigative results, X-rays (if applicable), medical notes and any other medical information required, to discuss with the consultant.

• During ward rounds, HOs discuss with consultants the patient's medical developments and any future plans of action required.

Senior House Officers (SHOs)

• Fully registered doctors who have completed 1 year of pre-registration (i.e. their names appear on the medical register).

• Can work independently, and do not have to be supervised to make management decisions, but are still accountable to consultants.

• Train pre-registration doctors and help with the HOs' daily tasks.

• Take outpatient (O/P) clinics.

Specialist Registrars

• Undergo specialist training. Help and advise SHOs. Take O/P clinics.

Consultants

• Highest senior level. Specialize in a specific area. Take O/P clinics. Train specialist registrars, SHOs and HOs, and manage specific wards (where applicable).

NURSES

- Nurses are trained and experienced carers in medical matters concerning patients. They are able to carry out medical and surgical routines under the supervision of a doctor.

- In the UK, student nurses undergo a specified period of training in a hospital approved by the General Nursing Council and pass an examination before qualifying for registration with the UKCC (United Kingdom Central Council for Nursing, Midwifery and Health Visiting) as a registered general nurse (RGN).

- Clinical nurse specialists develop expertise in areas such as diabetes, respiratory complaints, stoma care, breast care, tissue viability, infection control, symptom control, pain management, palliative care and paediatrics.

- Healthcare assistants (HCA) help nursing staff with their daily tasks.

- Three examples of nursing shifts include: early (7.30 a.m. to 3.30 p.m.); late (1.15 p.m. to 9.00 p.m.); and night (8. 45 p.m. to 8.00 a.m.). These will vary, however, among different hospitals and wards.

- Patient care is normally shared among nurses, e.g. using colour-coded 'nursing teams', but there are many other nursing systems which may be used for managing patient care.

- Always speak to the specific nurse dealing with your patient and determine which nursing system(s) are being used.

MULTIDISCIPLINARY TEAM

- Commonly, you will see physiotherapists, speech and language therapists, occupational therapists, social workers (the latter two being especially important in the community setting), podiatrists, pharmacists and radiographers involved in patient care.

Medical Records

MEDICAL NOTES—AN OVERVIEW

- A patient will enter hospital via Accident and Emergency (A&E), i.e. unexpected or acute urgency admission, or via their GP/consultant, i.e. a planned admission for either further tests or an operation.

- Planned admissions involve the GP writing a letter to an appropriate consultant, explaining the patient's medical problem and asking them for their medical/surgical opinion. A copy of this letter is normally kept at the back of the patient's hospital medical notes and is useful to look at for a summary of the patient's medical background and current condition.

- If the patient is referred via A&E, this will normally be documented with the patient's details and provisional diagnosis at the front of the hospital medical notes.

- Patients therefore have two separate medical notes, one held at the GP's practice and one at the hospital.

- Medical notes are divided into logical sections: commonly, current medical documentation at the front, and previous medical documentation (sectioned according to consultant or medical speciality), correspondence and investigations at the back.

- Inpatient's medical notes will be stored in a trolley at ward level, which will be in use during ward rounds (investigative results may also be held on hospital ward computers).

- Many wards are moving away from separate patient records, using integrated patient records instead (i.e. combining medical, nursing and professions allied to medicine records together).

- Internet access, in hospitals, via NHS-NET is a move towards a paper-free system with scope to access medical information throughout the UK and worldwide, e.g. medical journals, medical internet sites, NHS hospital information.

MEDICAL NOTES—CONTENT OUTLINE

When a patient is newly admitted, a full medical examination by an appropriate physician is undertaken. This consists of the following documentation:

- date admitted
- source of admittance (i.e. A&E, GP or consultant)
- present condition (PC)
- past medical condition (PMC) or past medical history (PMH), usually a dated list of previous medical conditions
- social history (SH), i.e. genetic, inherited factors, what parents died of (if applicable), type of housing/social support and present employment
- drug history (DH), i.e. drugs prescribed previously or currently to the patient or any known drug allergies
- complaining of (CO) present symptoms
- general examination (chest, respiratory function, muscular and bone movement)
- plan of action (tests ordered, referral to professions allied to medicine, etc.).

From here on, plans of action decided by doctors will be dated and briefly written in the patient's medical notes during ward rounds.

NURSING RECORDS

- Nurses may use a separate written system or 'integrated patient notes' (unitary records) for documenting patient's details.
- If unitary records are not used, nursing care plans may be kept in one main folder or separate folders for each patient. This will vary, however, among different wards and hospitals.
- Each patient will have a documented nursing care plan.

- Nursing care plans record patient's details, medical conditions/ treatment and nursing care. Daily nursing reports, for each patient, will be documented in these notes.

- It is useful to record in the nursing records a brief outline of your dietetic assessment and recommendations for a patient, so that during 'change-over', nurses have a written record to refer to.

DIETETIC DEPARTMENT RECORDS

- Dietetic department records vary in style and size but fundamentally record similar patient details.

- These records may be colour coded according to dietetic speciality, e.g. diabetes, renal or paediatrics, but this will vary among different departments.

- Patient's details recorded may include: blood biochemistry, weight, height, BMI, fluid balance, bowel movement, patient's wellbeing/social support, increased/decreased mobility, tests/investigations, diet history and dietary advice (as well as basic information such as the patient's name and home address).

- These details will be reviewed and documented where appropriate to assess any changes which may affect dietary intake.

- When a patient is discharged from hospital, document the discharge date and whether an O/P or any other follow-up appointment is required.

- Dietitians may use dietetic records to complete 'statistical records'. Statistical records are increasingly being used in hospitals to obtain specific data, e.g. monthly totals and types of patients seen by individual departments.

- The information gathered from statistical records may be used, in part, for audit purposes.

- Audits are a means of qualitatively and quantitatively measuring the effectiveness of a system or service, e.g. at departmental or ward level. Although as a student you may not be directly involved with clinical audit, it is important to be aware of this area. For further information refer to BDA (2000b).

- For information on record-keeping standards, refer to BDA (1996).

DIETETIC DOCUMENTATION IN THE MEDICAL NOTES

Dietitians have their own styles for recording dietetic information in the medical notes, and by the end of placement you will have developed your own. There are no right or wrong ways, but bear in mind the following guidelines:

- Always date and sign your entry, stating designation, i.e. 'student dietitian'.
- Always begin with 'thank you for referral....' for newly referred patients. This is considered good manners and hospital etiquette.
- You are legally required to use black ink.
- Write clearly and legibly.
- Use correct spelling.
- Avoid dietetic abbreviations (they may be misinterpreted by medical staff).
- Document information concisely.
- Never use correction fluid.

Here are two examples of recording a new dietetic referral for a 79-year-old female inpatient with malnutrition and chronic obstructive pulmonary disease (COPD).

EXAMPLE 1

Date seen by Student Dietitian

Thank you for referral of this 79-year-old malnourished woman with COPD.

Assessment	**Requirements**
Height: 1.5 m	1700 kcal/d
Weight: 55 kg	50–60 g protein/d
BMI: 18	

Patient reports weight loss of 3 kg over the past month. Owing to her tiredness and drowsiness, she is currently managing <600 kcal and 30 g protein daily.

Recommendations

1 2–3 × 300 ml high-energy/protein milk-based nutritional supplements/d (providing total 900 kcal, 35 g protein).

2 High-energy and protein foods ordered.

3 Small frequent meals/snacks.

To review food intake and weight.

Signature
(Student Dietitian)

EXAMPLE 2—SOAP GUIDELINES

Date seen by Student Dietitian

Subjective
Thank you for referring this 79-year-old woman with malnutrition and COPD. Owing to her tiredness and drowsiness, she is currently managing <600 kcal/d and 30 g protein daily.

Objective

Height: 1.5 m	Weight: 55 kg	BMI: 18

Current nutritional intake: energy <600 kcal/d; protein ~30 g/d

Assessment
Insufficient dietary intake to meet nutritional requirements. BMI of 18 suggests that this patient is moderately protein and energy depleted.

Plan

2–3 × 300 ml high-energy/protein milk-based nutritional supplements/d (providing total 900 kcal, 35 g protein) to be encouraged. Suitable high-energy/protein meals have been ordered. I feel that this patient would benefit from having small frequent meals/snacks. I have encouraged this and will continue to monitor the patient's progress, regularly.

Signature

(Student Dietitian)

For reviews or follow-ups, briefly outline any progress or changes in dietary prescription and date/sign entry.

Dietetic Referral Procedures

DIETETIC REFERRAL FOR A NEW INPATIENT— EXAMPLE CHECKLIST OF PROCEDURES

- Check dietetic referral in medical notes or on a referral form (it is unethical to see the patient otherwise, although some wards, e.g. an intensive care unit (ITU), may use a 'blanket' referral scheme, i.e. the ITU dietitian will automatically assess and review any patient(s) who require dietetic input).

- Read through medical/nursing records and discuss with appropriate nurse/referrer.

- Document relevant details on dietetic cards (e.g. patient's name, home address, GP, past medical history, present condition, social history, biochemistry and reason for dietetic referral).

- Document bed-end folder details into dietetic cards (e.g. present weight, height, bowel movements, temperature, fluid balance, medication, blood sugars, nutritional supplements and nasogastric feeding regimens, if applicable).

- Interview patient (liaise with relatives if appropriate/ available), and record information on dietetic records. (Refer to Appendix 3 for details on dietetic patient interviews.)

- Add relevant dietetic information to bed-end folder/nursing records (e.g. summary of assessment and recommendations, nasogastric feeding regimen, meal plans, food intake charts or special dietary instructions for medical staff to follow).

- Document dietary assessment and recommendations in medical/nursing records.

- Speak to the nurse looking after your patient, discussing with them the advice you have given to the patient.

- Follow up as required, depending on the patient's individual requirements and hospital dietetic review protocols.

Time Allowance for Referral

- 30–40 min per new inpatient (actual time spent will depend on available time and type of patient).

Follow Up Inpatient—Checklist

- Check medical/nursing records and liaise with medical staff/relatives.
- Check how the patient is getting on with food intake.
- Diet history (if required/time permits).
- Deal with any patient queries and encourage previous/new dietary recommendations.
- Inform the patient when you will next visit.
- Conclude interview.

Time Allowance for Follow-up

- 15–20 min per follow-up.

OUTPATIENTS (O/P)—AN OVERVIEW

- Once patients are discharged from hospital, they will be followed up as required, e.g. in O/P clinics. Alternatively, patients may be referred to dietetic O/P clinics via their GP or consultant.
- If you are seeing a new O/P, aim to record the patient's details from the medical notes into the dietetic records before seeing the patient, i.e. ideally obtain the medical notes pre-clinic.
- Obtain dietetic cards for review patients before a clinic starts (this will save time during a clinic).
- Normally, a dietitian will send a letter, outlining dietary assessment and recommendations, to the referring GP or consultant once the patient has been seen.
- Letters will also be sent to the referring GP or consultant if a patient fails to attend an appointment or is discharged from dietetic care.
- If medical notes are present, a brief dietetic summary should be documented.

Time Allowance

- 20–30 min new O/P.
- 10–15 min follow-up.

General Considerations

- Ensure that you keep up to date with recent developments of your patient, i.e. by checking medical notes and speaking to medical staff.
- Document all follow-up details in the dietetic cards and medical notes, e.g. weight changes, dietary assessments.
- As an outcome of most patient interviews, it is likely you will need to liaise with health professionals other than doctors and nurses, e.g. occupational therapists for eating implements, physiotherapists to schedule an enteral tube feed around a patient's daily exercise plan, and social workers to arrange 'meals on wheels' when a patient is discharged.

Dietetic Case Studies

- Case studies demonstrate the individual's ability to retrieve, interpret and utilize patient information to plan and carry out a treatment.

- For content and style of case studies, follow the practice of your base trainer. Most base trainers will have copies of previous students' case studies for you to look at. Refer to Dietitians' Board (2000) and Dietitians' Board/BDA (1991) for further information.

- Although you may do several smaller case studies (and present some of them), the main case study will have a content similar to the following outline.

EXAMPLE CONTENT OUTLINE FOR A MAIN CASE STUDY

- Patient's details (front cover): case x, sex, age, height (in metres), weight (in kg, e.g. pre-admission and discharge or before/after operation, include BMIs), ideal weight, medical diagnosis.

- Contents and appendices (new page).

- Acknowledgements (new page).

- Summary (new page), history of patient's symptoms and diagnosis.

- Social information: patient's age, gender, marital status and number of children, occupation, religious beliefs, type of living accommodation, kitchen storage, meal patterns (e.g. type of food eaten, who cooks, if patient eats out). Patient's views on nutrition.

- Past medical history (summarize).

- Recent medical investigations (summarize).

- Medical treatment, e.g. description of surgical/oncology treatments.

- Relevant drugs and their role (summarize).

- Involvement of other professions and their role (e.g. professions allied to medicine, social workers, clinical nurse specialists).
- Dietary treatment: describe in detail patient's dietary treatment, including biochemistry monitoring factors, calculation of nutritional requirements, weights, etc.
- Dietetic follow-up (summarize).
- Conclusion.
- Medical abbreviations (new page).
- Glossary (new page).
- References (new page).
- Bibliography (new page).
- Appendices (new page).

REFERENCES

British Dietetic Association (2000a)
NHS clinical dietetic placements: guidance for students on the allocation process. Birmingham: British Dietetic Association. Online: http://www.bda.uk.com

British Dietetic Association (2000b)
Dietitians and audit: a career long challenge. Birmingham: British Dietetic Association.

British Dietetic Association (1996)
Guidance for standards on records and record keeping. Birmingham: British Dietetic Association and the Dietitian's Board.

Byrne V (2000)
A day in the life: preparation for working in dietetics. Issue 1. News views talk in nutrition. London: ISIS.

Dietitians' Board (2000)
Pre-registration education and training. Birmingham: Dietitians' Board.

Dietitians' Board/British Dietetic Association (1991)
Student training resource pack. Birmingham: Dietitians Board.

DIETETIC
PATIENT
INTERVIEW

NOTES

- Appendix 3 outlines a dietetic patient interview for a newly referred inpatient intended to be used by dietitians. Relevant reference tables have been included.

- The taking of a 24-h diet history, described here, is outlined very simply, based on an inpatient having three set meals a day. In practice, this will vary greatly and therefore requires individual adaptation.

- As the information contained in this section is not comprehensive and is likely to vary among different dietetic departments, always follow the practice of your base trainer or own department.

- Information contained here will interlink with parts of Appendix 2, e.g. dietetic referral procedures, documenting dietetic information (refer to Appendix 2 for further details).

- There are many other techniques and sources of information available for patient interviewing and the taking of diet histories. For further information, refer to British Dietetic Association (1979), Bishop & Anthony (2001), Gable (1997) and Hollis & Calabrese (1997).

DIETETIC INTERVIEW—EXAMPLE CONTENT OUTLINE FOR A NEWLY REFERRED INPATIENT

1. Introduce Yourself to the Patient

- For example: 'Hello, my name is Jane Smith, I am a student dietitian. I hear/understand you've been having problems with …' (establish that your perception of the 'dietary problem' is the same as the patient's).

2. Explain the Interview Content to the Patient
(to help put the patient at ease)

- Explain that you are going to establish the patient's weight history and food intake to adapt dietary advice.

3. Establish the Patient's Weight History—Ask the Following:

- What is the patient's height?
- What is the patient's weight? (establish BMI)
- Has the patient always been this weight?
- When did the patient gain/lose this weight?

4. Establish the Patient's Recent Dietary Intake

Diet History (24-h recall)—Ask the Patient:

- What did the patient eat/drink first thing?
- What did the patient eat/drink for breakfast/lunch/evening meal?
- Did the patient eat/drink anything between these meals?
- Did the patient eat/drink anything mid-evening/before going to bed?
- Did the patient have any food/drink brought in by friends/relatives?
- Has the patient had any nutritional supplements?
- Has the patient had anything to eat/drink from the hospital shop/trolley?

(Alternatively, ask what the patient ate 'next' instead of using set mealtimes.)

During the 24-h Diet History, Aim to Establish:

- Quantities of food eaten.
- Composition of food eaten, e.g. 'full-fat', 'low-sugar' varieties.
- Time when food was eaten (especially relevant for patients with diabetes).
- When a patient last ate, if the patient has not eaten for the past 24 h, e.g. for patients who have been nil by mouth (NBM) for tests or operations.
- Eating/digestive problems (e.g. dysphagia, diarrhoea, constipation, nausea).

- Specific foods (if any) causing problems.
- Food preferences.
- Current carers (if any) bringing in 'favourite foods'.

5. Summary and Plan of Action

- Summarize to the patient main points gathered from the above information.
- Adapt and explain to the patient the meal plan/dietary advice.
- If applicable, let the patient try nutritional supplements (to distinguish taste preferences).
- Ask if the patient has any further questions.
- Let the patient know when you will next visit.
- Give thanks to the patient for their time and cooperation.
- Conclude interview.

NB: Interviews may not follow this order exactly. However, it is more important to obtain the relevant information and ensure that the patient understands and is able to follow the dietary advice given.

GENERAL CONSIDERATIONS

- Always establish with ward staff what patients know about their medical conditions before interviewing them. Some patients may not know their diagnoses yet or choose not to know.
- Treat each patient as an individual.
- Listen to the patient and aim to be as empathetic and understanding as possible.
- Avoid writing excessive notes during interviews (let the patient see you are actively listening).
- Be aware of a patient's physical and emotional condition. If you feel that it is inappropriate to see a patient or continue an interview, arrange another interview some time later. Inform and discuss the situation with ward staff, who may

be able to help during the interim, e.g. by offering the patient nutritional supplements.

- Some patients, especially chemotherapy patients, will have irregular eating patterns. Aim to establish dietary intake for days when they manage to eat well and days when they have difficulty eating.

- Be aware of the side-effects of certain medications which could cause nausea, vomiting and diarrhoea (see Section 3).

- Avoid jargon. Ask patients to recall dietary goals/advice to ensure that they have understood you (write down main points for the patient to reinforce this).

USEFUL DIET HISTORY/FOOD ABBREVIATIONS

A

alc/ETOH	Alcohol		

B

BE	Boiled egg	bp	Butter pat
BF	Breakfast	BU	Build up
Bix/bis/bic/bisc	Biscuits		

C

cc or cr	Cream crackers	Cot	Cup of tea
CF	Cornflakes	C.P.	Cheese portion
Choc	Chocolate	Chix	Chicken
coc	Cup of coffee		

D

DC	Double cream	Dig bi	Digestive biscuit
DM	Diabetic		

E

EM	Evening meal		

F

FE	Fried egg	FF	Full fat
FCM	Full cream milk	FJ	Fruit juice

G

g	grams	Gfr	Grapefruit
GF	Gluten free		

H

HP	High protein	HF	High fibre
HEP	High energy protein		

I
IC — Ice cream

J
Jkt — Jacket (potato)

K
Kcal — Calories · kg — Kilograms

L
L — Lunch · Low cal — Low calorie
LFS — Low-fat spread · lb — Pounds

M
Marg — Margarine · ml/s — millilitre/s
M/F — Meat/Fish · MP — Milk puddings
MK — Main kitchen · MW — Microwave

O
OJ — Orange juice · oz — Ounces

P
PE — Poached egg · Pudd — Pudding
Pot — Potato · pb — Plain biscuits
Porr — Porridge · Pt. — Pint

R
R.K. — Rice Krispies · Rst/R — Roast

S
Sat — Saturated fat · SMP — Skimmed milk powder
SE — Scrambled egg
S/W or S'wich — Sandwich · Supps — Supplements
S.S. — Semi-skimmed · STF — Sweet tinned fruit
SF — Sugar free · SVD — Sieved
x SMP — Supplemented milk pudding

T
Tin — Tinned · txd/liq — turmix/liquidized
Toms — Tomatoes

V
Veg — Vegetables

W
W'bix — Weetabix · W/M — Wholemeal
W/E — Weekend

Mealtimes

BF/B'fast — Breakfast · PM — Afternoon
MM — Mid-morning · EM — Evening meal
AM — Morning · S/Supp — Supper
L — Lunch · BB — Before bed
MA — Mid-afternoon

Table A3.1 Adult food portion sizes for 'common' foods

Food	Weight[a]
Pasta, noodles, pasta shapes (uncooked)	85 g (3 oz)
Rice (uncooked)	55–85 g (2–3 oz)
Potatoes (approximately 3–4 medium sized)	225 g (8 oz)
White fish	170–225 g (6–8 oz)
Roast beef	170 g (6 oz)
Minced beef	110–170 g (4–6 oz)
Beef steak	170–225 g (6–8 oz)
Stewing steak	110–170 g (4–6 oz)
Chicken breast	170–225 g (6–8 oz)
Roast pork	225 g (8 oz)
Pork or gammon steak	170 g (6 oz)
Butter/margarine (per serving on one slice of bread)	10 g (0.3 oz)
Hard cheese, e.g. cheddar (1-inch cube)	30 g (1 oz)
One medium slice of bread	25–30 g (1 oz)
One medium egg	50 g (1.6 oz)
One medium apple	75 g (2.5 oz)
One packet of crisps	28 g (1 oz)
One medium chocolate bar	54 g (1.8 oz)

[a]Approximate adult food portion sizes and weights; adapt to the individual.

Table A3.2 Nutritional composition of 'common' foods

Food	Portion size (g)	Energy kJ (kcal)	Protein (g)
Whole milk	100	271 (65)	3.3
Semi-skimmed	100	188 (45)	3.4
Skimmed	100	137 (33)	3.4
Yoghurt			
natural	150	351 (84)	7.7
fruit	150	564 (135)	6.2
One egg	60	367 (88)	7.5
One portion butter	10	376 (90)	0

Table A3.2 Nutritional composition of 'common' foods—continued

Food	Portion size (g)	Energy kJ (kcal)	Protein (g)
One slice hard cheese	40	689 (165)	10
Cream			
double	35	656 (157)	0.6
single	35	288 (69)	0.9
Ice-cream	75	610 (146)	2.7
One slice bread	25	229 (55)	2.2
Cornflakes	30	459 (110)	3.0
Two cracker biscuits	15	292 (70)	1.0
Sweet biscuits	15	292 (70)	1.0
Chicken, roast	85	769 (184)	20.0
Beef, roast	85	555 (133)	25.0
Beefburger, fried	60	668 (160)	12.0
Two sausages, grilled	90	1003 (240)	12.0
Fish			
in batter	130	1086 (260)	21.0
baked	120	501 (120)	22.0
Tuna in fish oil	95	1149 (275)	22.0
Rice boiled	165	836 (200)	3.6
Pasta boiled	150	652 (156)	5.4
Potato			
boiled	150	501 (120)	2.0
roast	130	852 (204)	3.5
fried	130	1379 (330)	5.0
Tomato, raw	60	83 (20)	0
Carrots, boiled	65	50 (12)	0.5
Apple	120	175 (42)	0
Banana	135	263 (63)	1.0
Orange	200	217 (52)	1.2
Sugar, two teaspoons	10	167 (40)	0
Chocolate	50	1107 (265)	4.2
Crisps	25	585 (140)	2.0
Peanuts	30	714 (171)	7.3

Source: Compositional data from McCance & Widdowson (2001).

Table A3.3   Energy content of 'common' alcoholic beverages

Classification	Beverage	Energy kJ (kcal)
Beers, lager and cider	Half-pint (284 ml) of:	
	Bitter	376 (90)
	Brown ale	334 (80)
	Light or mild ale	292 (70)
	Ordinary-strength lager	355 (85)
	Low-alcohol lager	250 (60)
	Dry cider	397 (95)
	Sweet cider	459 (110)
Spirits	One pub measure	
	(25 ml or 1/6 gill) of:	209 (50)
	brandy, whisky, gin,	
	rum or vodka	
Wine	Average glass size (113 ml) of:	
	Dry, white or red	313 (75)
	Sweet wine	418 (100)
	Rose	355 (85)
Sherry	One pub measure	
	(50 ml or 1/3 gill) of:	
	Dry	229 (55)
	Medium	250 (60)
	Cream	292 (70)
Mixers, soft drinks	Ordinary tonic	146 (35)
	Low-calorie tonic	0 (0)
	Can of coke	543 (130)
	Can of diet coke	0 (0)
	Glass of orange juice	334 (80)

Source: Compositional data compiled from McCance & Widdowson (2001).

APPENDIX 3

REFERENCES

Bishop JA, Anthony H (2001)
Student training education and practice in dietetics (Step Diet), 1st edn. CD-ROM. Surrey: University of Surrey. Online: http//:www.surrey.ac.uk/SBS/research/nutrition.htm

British Dietetic Association (1979)
Guidelines for taking diet histories. Birmingham: Working Party for the British Dietetic Association.

Gable J (1997)
Counselling skills for dietitians. Oxford: Blackwell Science.

Hollis BB, Calabrese RJ (1997)
Communication and education skills: the dietitians guide, 2nd edn. USA: Lippincott Williams and Wilkins.

McCance, Widdowson (2001)
The composition of foods, 5th edn. Cambridge: The Royal Society of Chemistry, Ministry of Agriculture, Fisheries and Food.